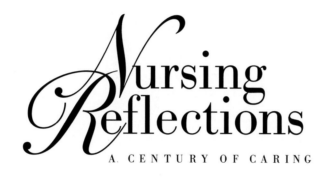

Nursing Reflections

A. CENTURY OF CARING

Nursing Reflections

A CENTURY OF CARING

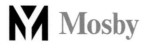

Mosby

A Harcourt Health Sciences Company

St. Louis   London   Philadelphia   Sydney   Toronto

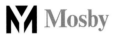

Mosby

A Harcourt Health Sciences Company

Editor-in-Chief Sally Schrefer
Executive Editor June D. Thompson
Senior Developmental Editor Linda Caldwell
Project Manager Carol Sullivan Weis
Project Specialist Pat Joiner
Design and Layout Amy Buxton
Cover photo provided courtesy of MedStar Health Visiting Nurse Association serving Washington, D.C., Maryland, and Northern Virginia.

Mosby, Inc.
A Harcourt Health Sciences Company
11830 Westline Industrial Drive
St. Louis, Missouri 63146

Printed in the United States

International Standard Book Number 0-323-01173-X

00 01 02 03 04 TG/KPT 9 8 7 6 5 4 3 2 1

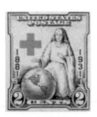

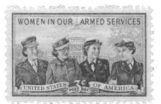

The year is 1970. The young father of five lay still on the bed in the ICU, his unscathed body belying the damage inside. His children, shepherded by 12-year-old Wendy carrying 1-month-old Patrick, come into the room hesitatingly, confused by the whooshing sound of the ventilator connected to his neck and their active father's quiet stillness. The nurses enter to do something, check something, talk to him and to the family. They've seen it before. The family dazed, unbelieving, hoping, praying; the patient's body trying to repair unfixable damage.

I watched the nurses, at first to see how my husband responded, and later when I began to allow myself to think the impossible–that he wouldn't survive–to marvel at their work, their words, their caring. Until those terrible days, I didn't know what all nurses did to take care of their patient, nor did I realize that they would take care of me, too.

My grandmother had been a nurse, graduating from Altmann Hospital School of Nursing in Canton, Ohio, in 1914. Her tales of the rigors of nurses' training were awe-inspiring and frightening. Twelve-hour days, seven days a week, with an occasional Sunday afternoon off if they weren't too busy and if it was to attend something to improve their minds or souls. One time, she told me, she and her classmates attended a revival meeting featuring the evangelist Billy Sunday. Coming back on the streetcar, they got off to transfer to another car and noticed an ice cream store at the corner. Dashing inside they hurriedly ordered their cones and rushed outside to find their streetcar had already left. When they returned to the hospital, they were severely scolded, and Sunday afternoons off were canceled for some time. Grandmother never forgot that responsibility to her patient came first.

She survived nurses' training and worked off and on all her life as a private duty nurse. She once said she had nursed many people to their death. As a child I feared becoming ill and needing her to "nurse" me. Later, I learned what compassion it took to care for the dying and to stay with them until the end. Now I was living it.

One night about 3 AM while I was sleeping on a sofa outside my husband's room, I heard his nurse talking to him. As she was ministering to his broken body, she talked about his family, his children, his wife, how much they loved him, cared about him, were waiting for him to get well. I lay there transfixed. She was talking to him as if he heard her even though he had been unconscious for more than a week! I, of course, talked to him all day as I sat by his bed, leaving only to eat, sleep, and breastfeed the baby when he was brought to the hospital. But the nurse didn't love him as I did. Then it dawned on me–she must care this much for all her patients. I decided then that if he did not recover, I would become a nurse, and I would help tell the world about what nurses really do. It is with pleasure I find this book that so beautifully illustrates nurses' caring, competence, compassion, and, most of all, their commitment to their patients.

When she learned I was attending nursing school, my grandmother, long since retired from nursing, gave me one piece of advice. "Just be a good nurse," she said, with a knowledgeable shake of her head. The nurses depicted here, and the millions they represent, understood.

Eleanor J. Sullivan, RN, PhD, FAAN
PROFESSOR
UNIVERSITY OF KANSAS SCHOOL OF NURSING
PAST PRESIDENT, SIGMA THETA TAU INTERNATIONAL

V

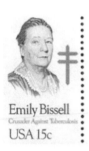

Emily Bissell
Crusader Against Tuberculosis

USA 15c

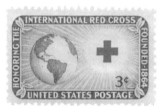

The Gift of Self

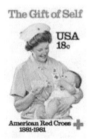

We live in an age awash in electronic and print images of people, places, and events, but to find a book devoted to photographs from the history of American nurses and nursing care is unusual. The reasons for this fact are simple. There were few photographs taken of nurses early in the century, and only a small number of these survived. One is able to find personal scrapbooks filled with photographs of student nurses celebrating such events as receiving their new uniforms and caps and graduating, but seldom found are photos of students or private duty nurses engaged in patient care in hospitals or homes. At the turn of the twentieth century the technical complexity and expense of photography, and the sense of impropriety of photographing patients, restricted the use of a camera in documenting the identity and role of nurses. Equally true was the fact that when hospitals began to use photography to inform the public of the scientific sophistication of their modern facilities and their expert physicians, nurses were not considered important factors in assuring the public and financial donors of the healing benefits of the hospital to the community.

A review of photos found in hospital advertisements and annual reports reveals not only the publicity benefit of the posed and artificial images but also the social hierarchies found among the hospital staff. Images of hospital wards, clinics, and surgical operating rooms portray a clean, white, and orderly environment, modern scientific equipment; and satisfied patients attended by skillful and knowledgeable physicians. Nurses may be found in these photos, but typically they are situated peripherally from the main activity depicted in the photograph. In addition, the nurses often look directly at the camera while the physicians focus their attention on caring for the patients.

Photographs of community health nurses, however, are more easily found than those of hospital nurses, and they portray nurses as solitary practitioners caring for needy patients in their homes. Sprinkled throughout visiting nurse agencies' annual reports are found posed photographs of nurses teaching or caring for mothers, babies, and children, as well as an occasional bed-ridden adult. Because visiting nurse agencies existed primarily through the financial generosity of donors, these official photographs depicted the social mission of community health nurses. This mission included caring for vulnerable families, and in doing so, nurses protected the health and future of the community.

By the 1950s, hospitals began to recognize that photographs of attractive nurses with patients, particularly mothers and children, generated a positive image of the care available in their institutions. The use of nurses to market the human caring quality of patient services struck a warm response among potential patients and financial donors. Soon, hospital reports, particularly those aimed for public consumption, were filled with photos of nurses as well as physicians and technology.

Regardless of the reasons that hospital or community health photographs were taken, each photo opens a unique window into nursing's past. The reader of this book will easily identify differences in nurses' uniforms, hospital architecture, medical technology, and nursing procedures over the century. However, setting these differences aside, the power of the photographs lay in their ability to capture similarities to today's nurses and patients. The images reaffirm not only the youth and vitality of previous generations of nurses but also their sense of caring and dedication to the care of the sick, the preservation of human life, and when that was not possible, the compassionate care of the dying.

Barbara Brodie, PhD, RN, FAAN
MADGE P. JONES PROFESSOR OF NURSING
DIRECTOR, CENTER OF NURSING HISTORICAL INQUIRY
UNIVERSITY OF VIRGINIA SCHOOL OF NURSING
CHARLOTTESVILLE, VIRGINIA

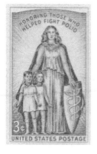

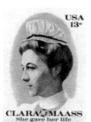

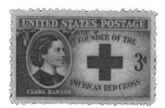

*I*t was 1893 when Nightingale wrote the following about "sick nursing and health nursing":

> A new art and a new science has been created since and within the last forty years. And with it a new profession–so they say; we say, calling. One would think this had been created or discovered for some new want or local want. Not so. The want is nearly as old as the world, nearly as large as the world, as pressing as life or death. It is that of sickness, and the art is that of nursing the sick. Please mark–nursing the sick; not nursing sickness. We call the art nursing proper.

And so, that was the stage set at the beginning of the twentieth century. The past 100 years have produced advances in nursing and health care that not even the wildest minds could have imagined. Throughout this century we have observed the discovery of blood types, antibiotics, vitamins, and vaccines. Hearts have been transplanted, and iron lungs, once used to support breathing, now rest in museums. We have conquered polio, eradicated smallpox, identified HIV and AIDS, and we continue to test new protocols to battle cancer.

We have participated as hospitals have expanded, specialized, upsized, and downsized. We have taken our care back into the homes, schools, migrant camps, community clinics, prisons, and similar community settings. We have learned of the benefits of Medicare and Medicaid and have watched the creation and demise of numerous new roles of health care specialties.

Nurses have been there throughout the century, responding to the needs of the nation. We have followed our troops around the world during times of war and distress; climbed on horseback to meet the needs of rural families; walked to migrant camps to care for workers; delivered babies in homes, in elevators, and on the lawn; run clinics in storefronts, churches, and community centers; responded to the needs of the ill or injured by learning to operate equipment, sometimes a lot of equipment; we have demonstrated over and over our advocacy for those for whom we care; and we have learned to finagle the system to help individuals and families get their health care needs met. Finally, and indeed most important, we have continued throughout the twentieth century to care, to share joy and sadness, and to continuously hold the hands and hearts of all those for whom we have provided care.

This photo essay book portrays the continual caring provided by nurses throughout the past century. As you look at the photos, review the timelines, and read the letters and notes from nurses, we hope you see and feel beyond the printed material and become absorbed in the multitude of contributions nursing has provided not only to individuals and families but also to society during the past century.

June D. Thompson, DrPH, RN
EXECUTIVE EDITOR
HARCOURT HEALTH SCIENCES

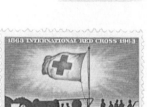

The editor is grateful for all those who have contributed to the richness of this book. Special thanks goes to the universities, hospitals, organizations, agencies, and individuals who have submitted photos and to the nurses who have shared stories from their own personal experiences.

INDIVIDUALS

Catherine Bane
Betty Ann Beaudry
Linda Bowers
Rick Brady
Barbara Brodie
Sandra Tebben Buffington
Karen Buhler-Wilkerson
Stuart Campbell
Mary Ann Draye
Evelyn B. Elder
Sister Marie G. Frigo
Sandra L. Gardner
Marian Louise Goff
Kathy Haley
Mary Martha Hall
Harriette Hartigan
Lena Hurst
Jill Johnson
Joan Kasson
Linda L. Larson
Mary Ann Lewis
Shirley A. Martin
Ethel Colcord Mattingly
Margaret M. McMahon
Pam Meredith
Pam Morgan
Katherine Priddy
Donna Proulx
Anna Marie Rutallie
Susan Sacharski
Eleanor J. Sullivan
Susan Swasta
Sister Jeanette Thelen
Juanita Mattingly Wagner
Ardis Wait
Betsy Weiss
Marti Whiting
Dolores Wright

INSTITUTIONS

American Heritage Center, University of Wyoming
Armed Forces Institutes of Pathology
Bascom Palmer Eye Institute
Center for Nursing Historical Inquiry, University of Virginia
Center for the Study of the History of Nursing, University of Pennsylvania
Frontier Nursing Service
Georgetown University School of Nursing Nurse Anesthesia Program
Hampton University Archives
Hutzel Hospital
Instructive Visiting Nurse Association of Richmond
Library of Congress
MedStar Health Visiting Nurse Association
Memorial Hermann Hospital Life Flight
National Archives and Records Administration
National Library of Medicine
Northwestern Memorial Hospital Archives
Rush-Presbyterian-St. Luke's Medical Center Archives
St. Vincent Health System
Villanova University College of Nursing
Visiting Nurse Association of Greater Philadelphia
Visiting Nurse Service of New York
University of California at Los Angeles School of Nursing
University of Texas School of Nursing Nurse-Midwifery Program
U.S. Air Force
U.S. Army Center of Military History
U.S. Army Military History Institute

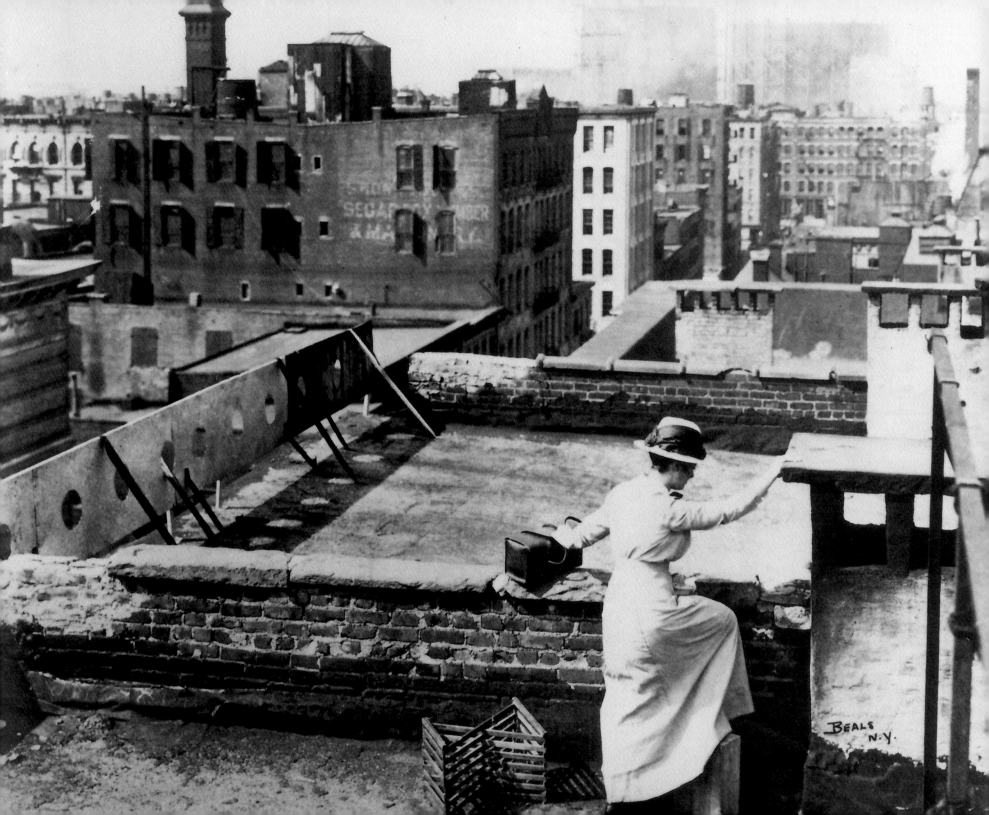

1900

The first automobile show is held in Madison Square Garden.

Sigmund Freud publishes *The Interpretation of Dreams*.

New Zealand passes the first Nurses' Registration Act, securing a mechanism to license the practice of nursing.

M. Adelaide Nutting begins the connection of higher education to nursing preparation by requiring students at Johns Hopkins University to complete 6-month basic sciences and nursing principles and practice courses before beginning experiences on the hospital wards.

Eastman Kodak introduces the $1 Box Brownie camera.

The bubonic plague breaks out in San Francisco.

A total of 1.5 million telephones are in use in the United States.

Major Walter Reed of the U.S. Army demonstrates the transmission of yellow fever from one human to another through the bite of the mosquito *A. aegypti*.

The first issue of the *American Journal of Nursing* is published.

1901

President McKinley is assassinated.

Guglielmo Marconi receives radio signals transmitted across the Atlantic.

Victoria, Queen of England and Empress of India, dies after reigning 64 years.

Karl Landsteiner discovers blood types.

The first electric typewriter, the Blickensderfer, is introduced.

1902

In New York City, Lillian Wald initiates public school nursing.

Willem Einthoven prints the first electrocardiograph recording on a string galvanometer.

In England, Sir William Bayliss and Ernest Starling discover secretin and coin the term *hormone*.

1903

California, New Jersey, New York, and Virginia become the first states to secure nursing licensure laws.

The Wright brothers make their first flight at Kitty Hawk, North Carolina.

1904

Alfred Einhorn develops Novocain, eliminating pain from most dental procedures and revolutionizing the practice of dentistry.

The Louisiana Purchase Exposition in St. Louis introduces the ice cream cone to the United States.

The telephone answering machine is invented.

1905

E. Zirm performs the first human corneal transplant.

The Yellow Pages are first published.

1906

An earthquake destroys many buildings and kills 2500 people in San Francisco.

Sir Frederick Hopkins discovers the amino acid tryptophan and later finds that it and certain other amino acids must be supplied in the diet; he terms the missing factors *vitamins*.

German physician August von Wasserman develops the test for syphilis.

1907

Oklahoma becomes the forty-sixth state.

A record 1.29 million immigrants enter the United States.

1908

Henry Ford's first Model T sells for $850.

The Provisional Organization of the Canadian National Association of Trained Nurses is formed; in 1924, the name is changed to the *Canadian Nurses Association*.

The National Association of Colored Graduate Nurses is established.

1909

The School of Nursing at the University of Minnesota becomes the first nursing school organized as an integral part of the university.

Congress passes the copyright law.

The National Negro Committee, later renamed the *National Association for the Advancement of Colored People (NAACP)*, is founded in New York.

1

2

The average ward ought to contain not more than twenty-five or thirty beds. The beds should be separated by a distance of at least three feet, and each patient should be allowed about sixteen hundred cubic feet of air space. For a ward of this size there should be not less than one bathroom, two closets, and if possible, one room set apart to contain nothing but the slop-hopper, racks for holding vessels, shelves for urine jars, and catheter bottles.

The head nurse of the ward, besides being a thoroughly trained nurse, should be a woman of executive ability, economical, and with some practical knowledge of housekeeping. She is held responsible for everything pertaining to the ward, and if the patients are only imperfectly cared for, the blame will not fall upon the assistant nurses so much as upon her.

Modified from NURSING: ITS PRINCIPLES AND PRACTICE, *J.B. Savage, Isabel Adams Hospital, Cleveland, Ohio*, 1901

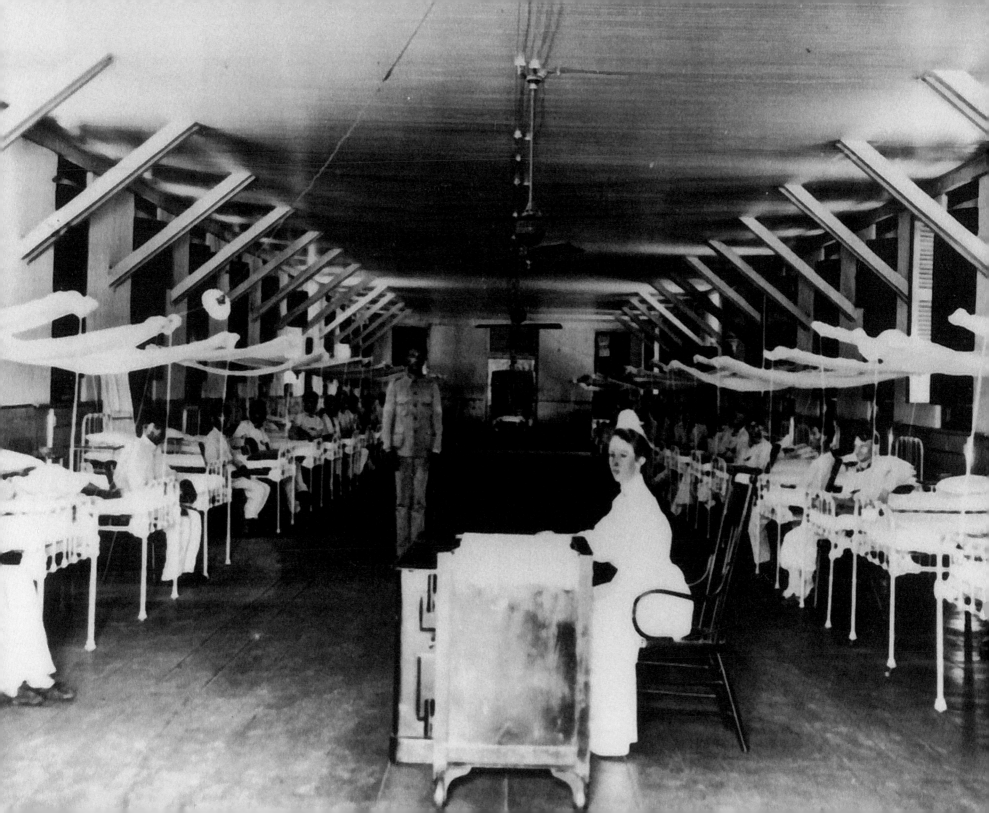

4

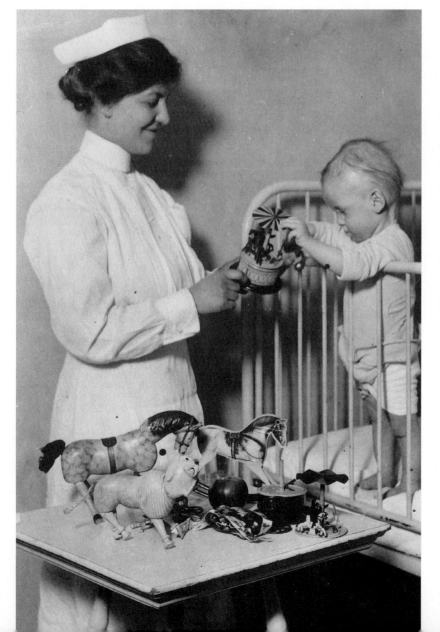

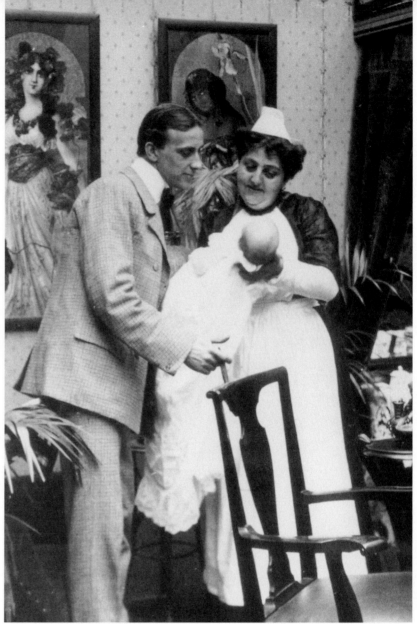

Caring: the art of having concern for others and protecting from harm.

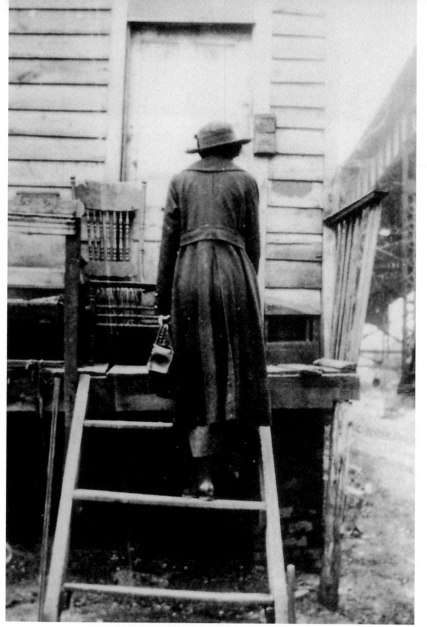

I hope Miss Taylor is feeling better today.

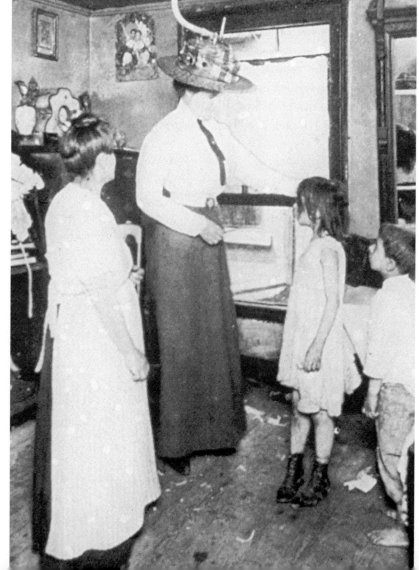

N urses provided care in the home to deliver the babies and check on the children from school.

ORDER OF WORK FOR NURSES

THE TEMPERATURE NURSE takes the temperatures and charts them; gives medicines and keeps the medicine-closet in order; makes out and gives daily to the head nurse the list of medicines to be replenished; gives out meals and special nourishment; and is responsible for the appearance of the kitchen.

THE NURSE ON THE RIGHT SIDE OF THE WARD cares for bed patients of that side, gets the convalescents up, makes the beds, does the dusting, and is responsible for the general good order of everything on that side. In addition, she keeps the linen-closet in order and folds the fresh linen.

THE NURSE ON THE LEFT SIDE OF THE WARD has the same duties as the nurse on the right side, and in addition is responsible for the bath-room and lavatory.

THE THIRD NURSE takes care of the special patients in the small rooms and looks after the dressing-carriage. She is also responsible for the preparation of patients for operations.

THE PROBATIONER, OR JUNIOR NURSE, assists in making beds and doing the dusting, carbolizes beds, cleans mackintoshes, lists soiled clothes for the laundry, lists and puts away new patients' clothes, and is responsible for the patients' clothes-closet. She also assists in giving out meals.

A nurse's manner toward her patient should be characterized always by a gentle dignity. She should be wisely sympathetic, and, while never familiar nor tolerant of the least familiarity, should always make the patients feel that they are her first consideration, and that to do anything for their comfort is her greatest pleasure.

There is nothing for a nurse to do but to go on steadily with her work: general conversation between nurses while in the ward is strictly forbidden; an occasional question regarding the work is all that is permissible. The same remarks apply to the nurse's relation to the hospital physicians. The ward is not the place, and "on duty" not the time, for indulging in social talk–the time belongs to the patients, and a right-minded, conscientious nurse will never permit her patients to be deprived of what is justly theirs.

Modified from NURSING: ITS PRINCIPLES AND PRACTICE, *J.B. Savage, Isabel Adams Hospital, Cleveland, Ohio*, 1901

6

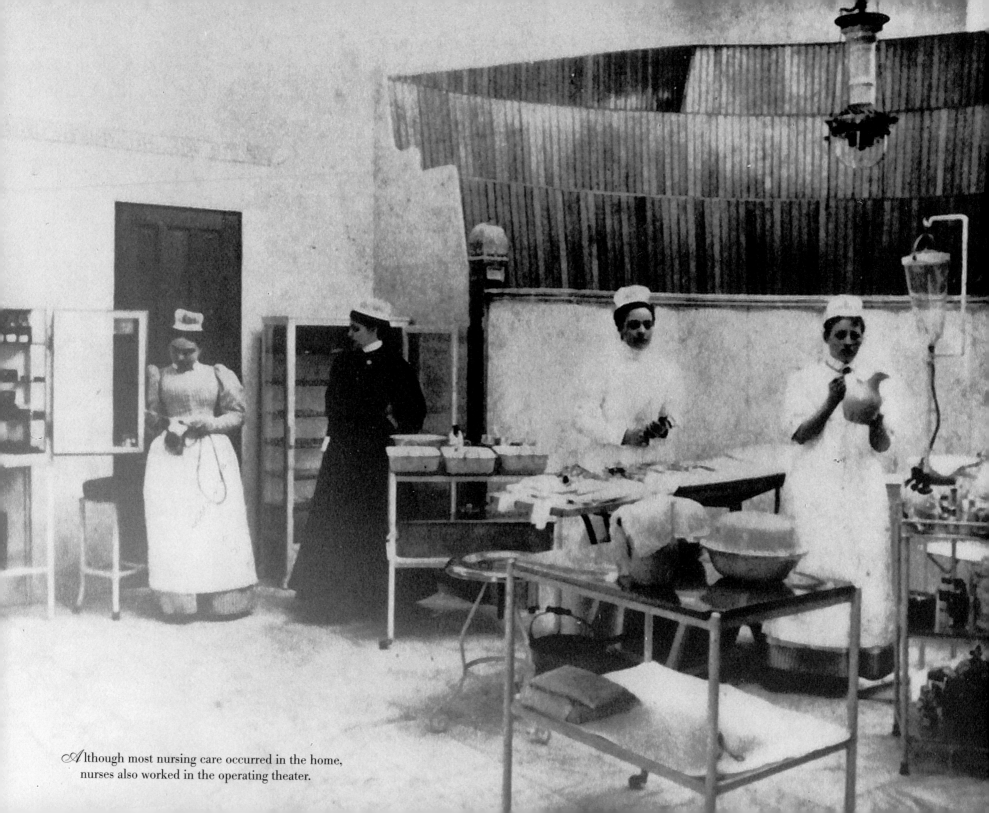

Although most nursing care occurred in the home, nurses also worked in the operating theater.

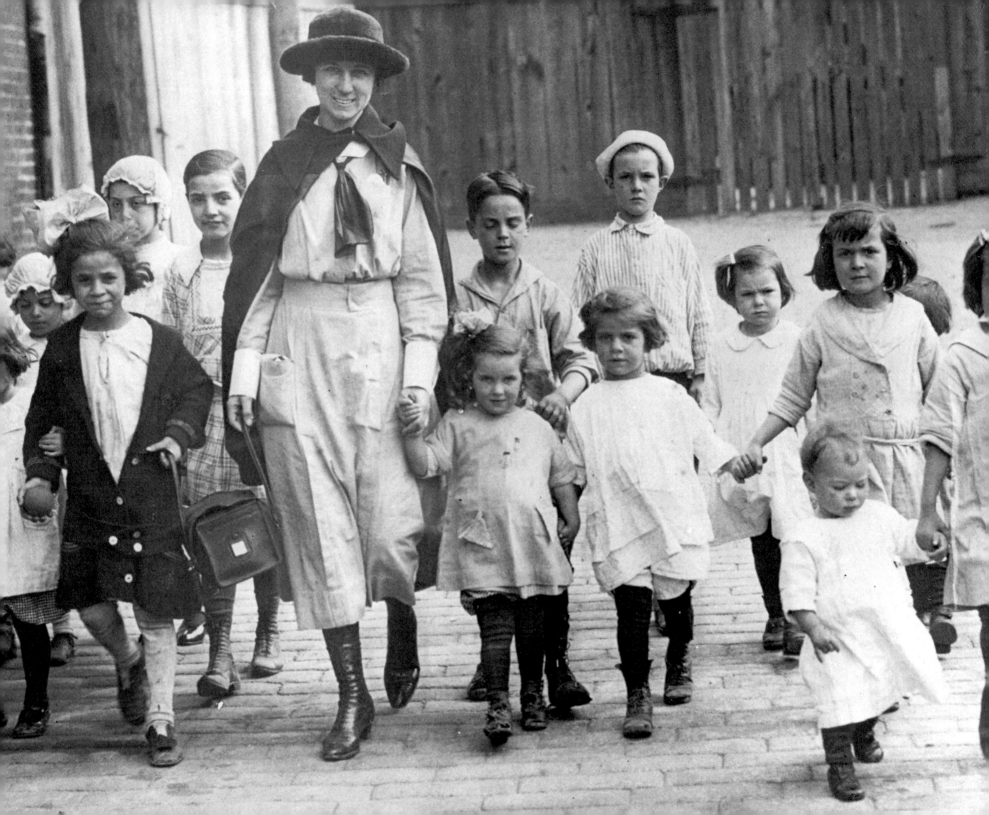

1910s

1910

In August, Florence Nightingale dies at the age of 90.

Halley's comet returns; it will next appear in 1986.

Writer Mark Twain dies.

1911

Bellevue Hospital establishes the first U.S. school of midwifery.

The American Nurses' Association becomes the successor to the Nurse's Associated Alumnae.

The first laparoscopy, called *organoscopy*, is conducted at Johns Hopkins University Hospital.

Ernest Rutherford discovers the nucleus of the atom.

A revolution in China ends the 267-year Qing dynasty.

1912

In April, the Titanic hits an iceberg and sinks; 1523 die.

Congress establishes the Children's Bureau to investigate the welfare of children and the child labor situation in America. Lillian Wald is credited with the idea of establishing this agency.

The American Society of Superintendents of Training Schools is renamed the *National League of Nursing Education*.

The National Organization for Public Health Nursing (NOPHN) is established.

New Mexico and Arizona join the Union as new states.

1913

Albert Schweitzer organizes a hospital in Lambaréné, Gabon, in Africa.

J. Abel, L.G. Roundtree, and B.B. Turner arrange a mechanical system they call an *artificial kidney*, whereby the blood of a dog could be freed of toxic chemicals by circulating it through collodion tubing that allowed toxins to pass out into surrounding liquid while keeping blood substances inside.

Congress institutes the personal income tax.

The R.J. Reynold's Company introduces the first cigarettes, Camel.

In Sarajevo, Austrian archduke Francis Ferdinand and his wife Sophie are assassinated, causing a chain reaction leading to World War I.

In August, the Panama Canal opens after 10 years of construction.

George Washington Carver's experiments with peanuts provide Southern farmers a new crop to grow after the boll weevil devastated the cotton industry.

1914

Long-distance telephone service is established between New York and San Francisco.

Margaret Sanger, a nurse working with poor women, coins the term *birth control* and opens a women's clinic in Lower New York City.

The cruise liner, Lusitania, on a journey from New York to Liverpool, is sunk by a German U-boat, killing almost 2000 people and contributing indirectly to the entry of the United States into World War I.

British nurse Edith Cavell is arrested in Brussels for helping British, French, and Belgian soldiers escape from behind German lines. Two months later, she is executed before a firing squad.

1915

New York's Teachers College and the University of Cincinnati are the first universities to establish 5-year bachelor-degree programs in nursing.

Albert Einstein publishes his "General Theory of Relativity."

1916

The United States enters World War I by declaring war on Germany.

The Bolshevik Party seizes power in Russia, leading to the execution of Tsar Nicolas and his family and the inauguration of the Soviet regime.

Mexican revolutionary "Pancho" Villa leads raids into New Mexico, killing 18 Americans. President Wilson orders U.S. troops under General John J. Pershing to pursue him, but Villa is never caught.

1917

President Wilson outlines his proposals for postwar peace in his "Fourteen Points."

World War I ends when the Armistice document is signed in a railway car near Rethondes, France.

An epidemic of the Spanish flu called the *doomsday flu* kills 20 million in Europe and Asia.

The United States establishes Grand Canyon and Acadia National Parks.

1918

Radio broadcasts begin.

The pandemic of influenza reaches the United States, causing approximately 500,000 deaths.

The dial telephone is introduced.

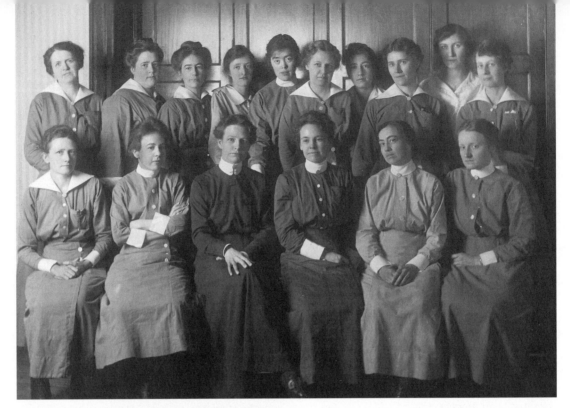

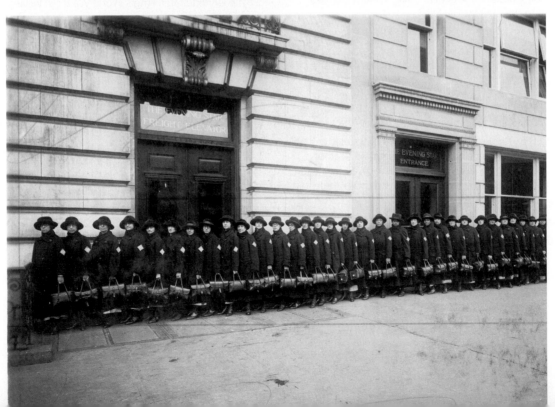

Nursing Ethics: Hospital conditions are not those of ordinary life. In nursing, we deal with the unusual and the abnormal.

Within the walls of the hospital we find that we must accept all people as they are, and devote ourselves mainly to their physical betterment. This is right because our dealings are only with the unusual. To accept people and conditions as they are and to do our best with them is our present business and needs our entire attention.

Nursing a Profession: The actual work done by a nurse can be learned by a person of ordinary intelligence; but the fine art of nursing is a thing which requires special fitness, special and long training, and determined application. We hear of the "born" nurse. There is no such person, though we may by courtesy apply the term to her who by her interest, enthusiasm, faithfulness, diligence, and loving spirit, puts the work of caring for the sick among the professions. She may have talent for nursing, as a painter or musician has talent for art or music, but she must, as they do, process the determination which makes her go through years of training in the technique and spirit of her art.

Qualities Requisite for a Nurse: Two of the qualities for which superintendents of training schools most often look in accepting a probationer are good breeding and teachableness. These produce the proper spirit, which is the foundation.

The Patient and Chief Consideration: The one fact which should never be lost sight of is the patient is the main thing. His welfare is the objective of the hospital's existence.

Military Discipline: The organization and discipline of the hospital resembles that of the army. Unquestioning obedience to superiors is expected.

Truthfulness: If a nurse makes a mistake, it is not only the honorable but the wise course for her to report it without delay.

Relations not Social: Especially must she remember that while on duty her relations to those about her are not social but professional.

Other employees: All orderlies, maids, cooks, and other employees are in a different class from the nurse, and any social intimacy is forbidden.

Visitors: Visitors who come into the hospital should be treated as you would the guests of a friend who is stopping with you.

Familiarity: Guard against familiarity with patients; it is always productive of untoward results.

Considerations: Be considerate. Do not insist upon your way, but whenever it is at all possible, permit a patient to do as he pleases.

Contradicting: Never contradict a patient's statement in his presence. If he says what you believe to be untrue, you can give your view of it when outside the sick-room.

Manner: Avoid a hurried manner: You may work quickly, but the moment a suggestion of haste creeps in, the keen eye of the patient interprets it as a lack of interest, which in truth it is, being plainly disregard for the matter in hand and seeking for something outside.

Distinction between Persons: Make no distinction between rich and poor, between attractive and unattractive persons.

Expression of Emotion: Train your face to express or not express emotion, as you will it. A nurse whose face is an open book is likely to be the occasion of much discomfort or even disaster.

Truthfulness with Patients: Be honest with your patient. Nurses commonly and all too quickly fall into the way of thinking that it is not only permissible but right to tell untruths to the patient.

The Nurse's Appearance: The nurse must make her personal appearance the subject of extreme care. Every moment of her time on duty she is on dress parade, every detail of her dress and bearing is subjected to inspection and criticism, and the patient's final judgment of her is made up of very small considerations.

Neatness: She must be neat to the point of immaculateness. Her dress must have no rip, no tear, no worn place, no frayed edge.

Spirit of the Work: In your work, be ready to do more than is expected of you. Consider your work as opportunity, and bear in mind that the harder it is the more training you are getting.

Quality of Work: Finally, let the quality of your work be your chief pride. Never be content with half-way or fairly good work. Make it your best. Let each task be a finished piece of work, each undertaking a model of neatness and orderliness. Then shall nursing be not hard work, but a fine art.

Modified from Minnie Goodnon, *W. B. Saunders Company, Philadelphia, Pennsylvania,* 1919

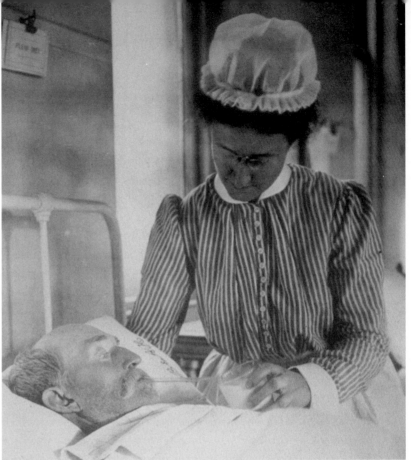

12

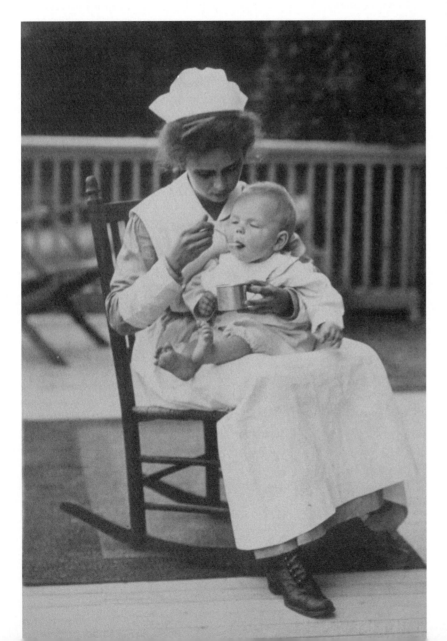

Caring: to pay close attention to...
          to provide watch over or to attend to...

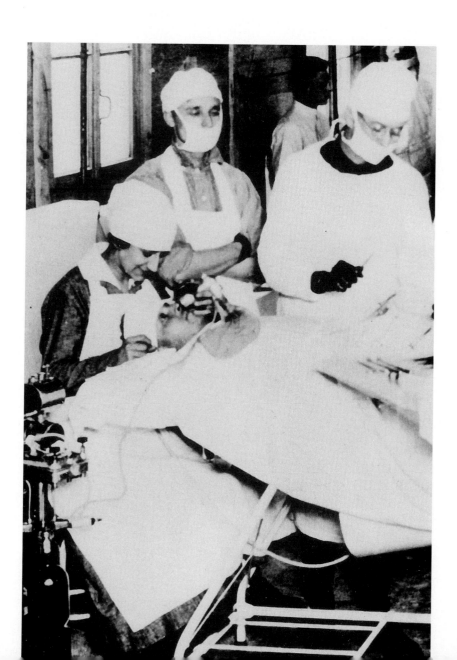

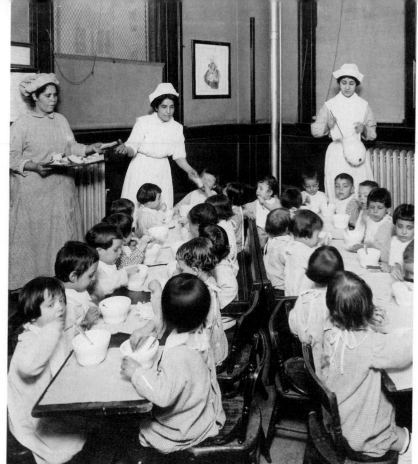

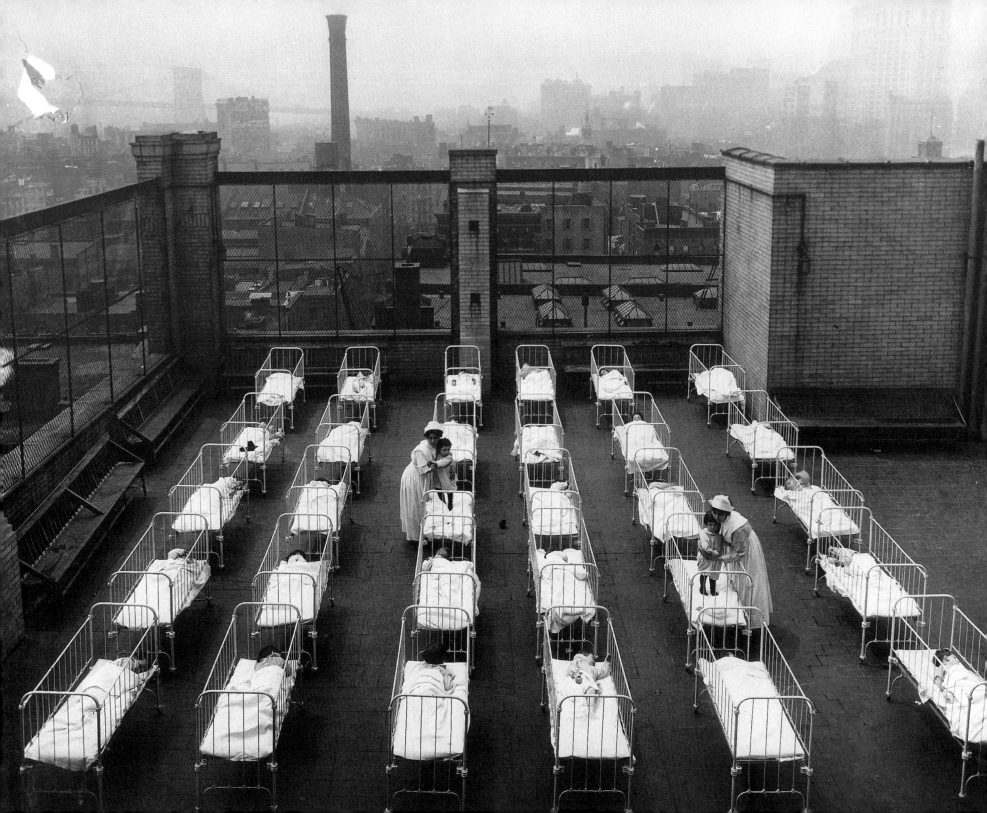

CLEANING, FUMIGATION, VENTILATION

"So clean that it cannot be cleaner."

IMPORTANCE OF CLEANLINESS: One of the first lessons a nurse must learn is that of scrupulous cleanliness. Ordinary household cleanliness is not sufficient in a hospital. In our homes we clean largely for the sake of appearance; in the hospital, cleaning is done for the safety of the patient.

COMPOSITION OF DUST: Hospital dust contains particles of dirt blown in from the street containing germs dropped by animals, etc., lint from the bedding, scales from the skin, dandruff from the head, dried throat and nasal secretions, particles of dried excreta, and many other substances both disagreeable and dangerous.

ARRANGEMENT OF THE WORK OF CLEANING: In private nursing, the nurse is personally responsible for the cleaning of her patient's room, and except in families where several servants are kept, is expected to do it herself. Servants are apt to annoy a sick person, and they rarely know how to clean properly. A maid cleans only for appearance's sake; a nurse cleans in accordance with the underlying scientific principles.

SWEEPING: Dry sweeping with a broom on bare floors is both unsanitary and ineffective. A soft bristle brush collects and removes more of the dust and does not scatter it into the air. Always begin to sweep the edge of the room, and work toward the center and toward the door.

WIPING FLOORS: After the bulk of the visible dirt is removed by one means or another, the floor should be wiped, so that any bacteria, which are far too small to be taken up by a dry process, may be caught on a damp surface and carried away.

CLEANING RUGS: Rugs should be hung on a line out of doors and beaten. A wicker beater is best, as a wire one cuts the threads. Rugs may be shaken, but shaking wears them out rapidly, soils the hands, hair, and clothing of the person who does it.

Many accidents to handsome rugs could be avoided if nurses would push them away from the bedside when they begin a douche, enemas, or surgical dressings. It takes but a moment to remove or to replace them while accidents are expensive and annoying.

DUSTING: Dusting in the hospital sense of the word means removing all dust from the room, not simply pushing it from one place to another. To be of any real use, it must be done with a damp cloth.

How TO DUST—begin with the dresser, chairs, and articles made of wood, having the cloth just damp enough to collect the dust. Everything on the dresser should be removed and each individual piece wiped off.

OBSERVATION: One of the marks of a good nurse is her ability to see things. This power can be cultivated from the first day in the hospital. If you cannot see a dirty spill on a table or a bedspread which is awry, you will hardly be able to recognize the fine points of change in a patient's condition which are so often important danger signals.

CARE OF PLANTS AND FLOWERS: Plants and flowers are usually set off the rooms or the wards during the night. After the morning dusting is done, they should be cared for and taken back to the patients. Remember that each plant or flower is an expression of some person's regard for another, and treat it with the care it deserves.

ARRANGING FLOWERS—do not be guilty of putting more than one sort of suitable size and shape. Get the stems well into the water, but not so far down as to spoil the effect of the arrangement.

WATERING PLANTS—potted plants with many blooms or broad leaves need a great deal of water. Azaleas and cyclamens in particular should be kept well soaked. Few things give a worse impression on than for a nurse to allow a beautiful plant to wither for want of water.

Modified from REGULATIONS FOR NURSES, *St. Francis Hospital, Hartford, Connecticut,* 1913

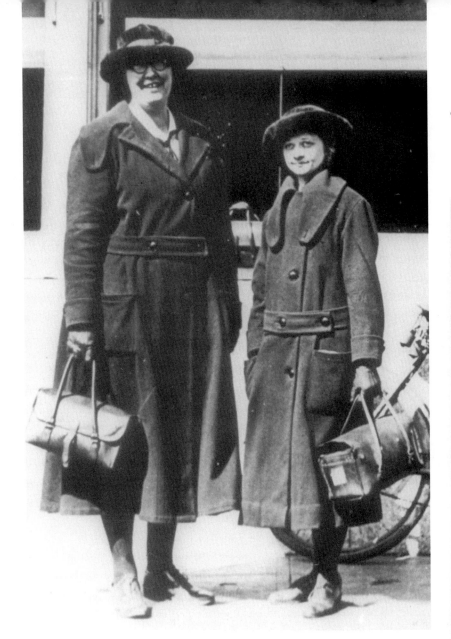

16

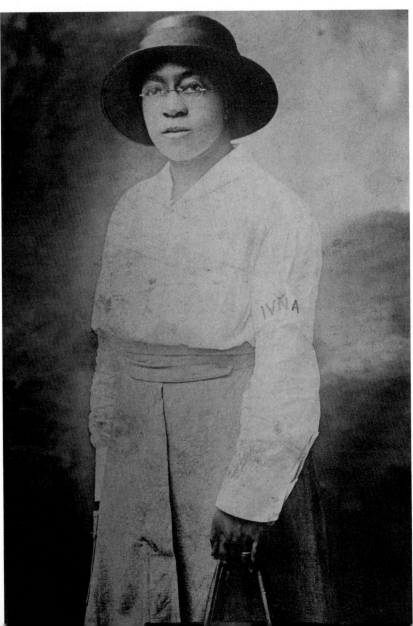

*Nurses were among the first to provide health care in the community...
in all types of communities.*

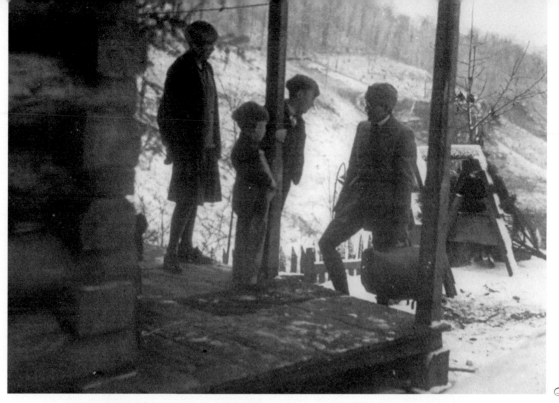

*M*aking home visits wherever they are needed.

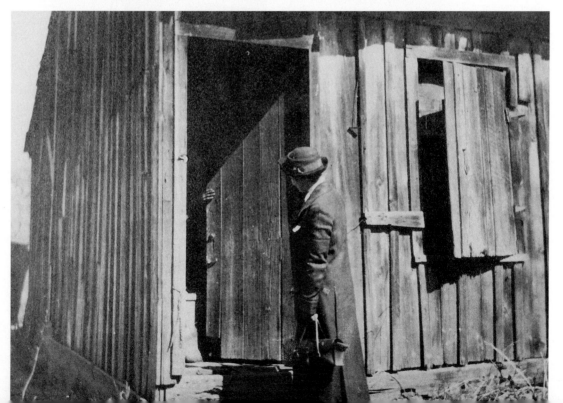

During World War I almost 23,000 graduate nurses served in Army and Navy cantonments and hospitals, and more than 10,000 served overseas. A total of 260 nurses died either in the line of war duty or because of the influenza epidemic.

At least 3 Army nurses were awarded the Distinguished Service Cross, the nation's second highest military honor. Several received the Distinguished Service Medal, the highest noncombat award, and over 20 were awarded the French Croix de Guerre.

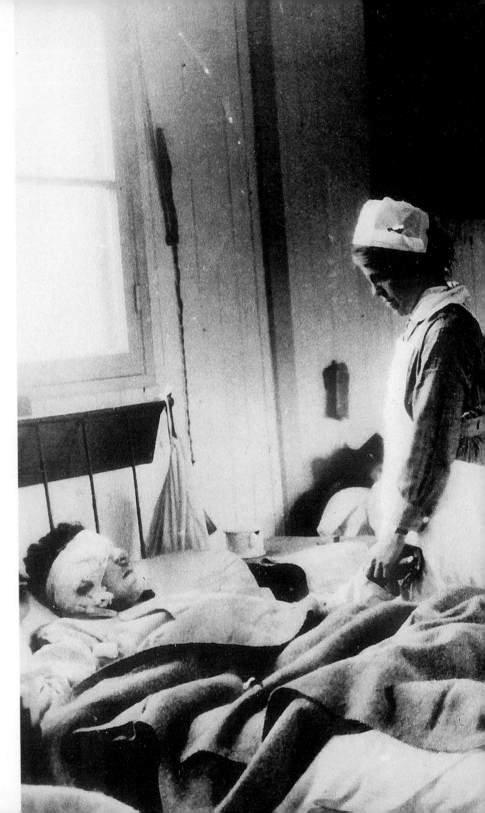

American Red Cross nurse in an evacuation hospital in France.

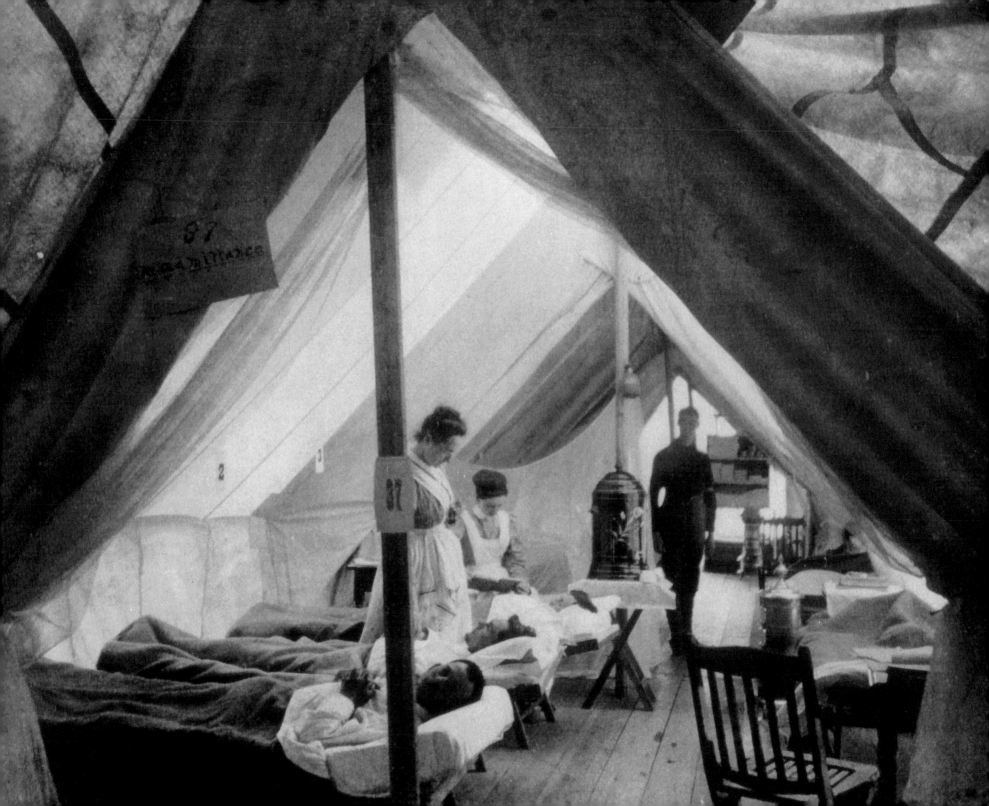

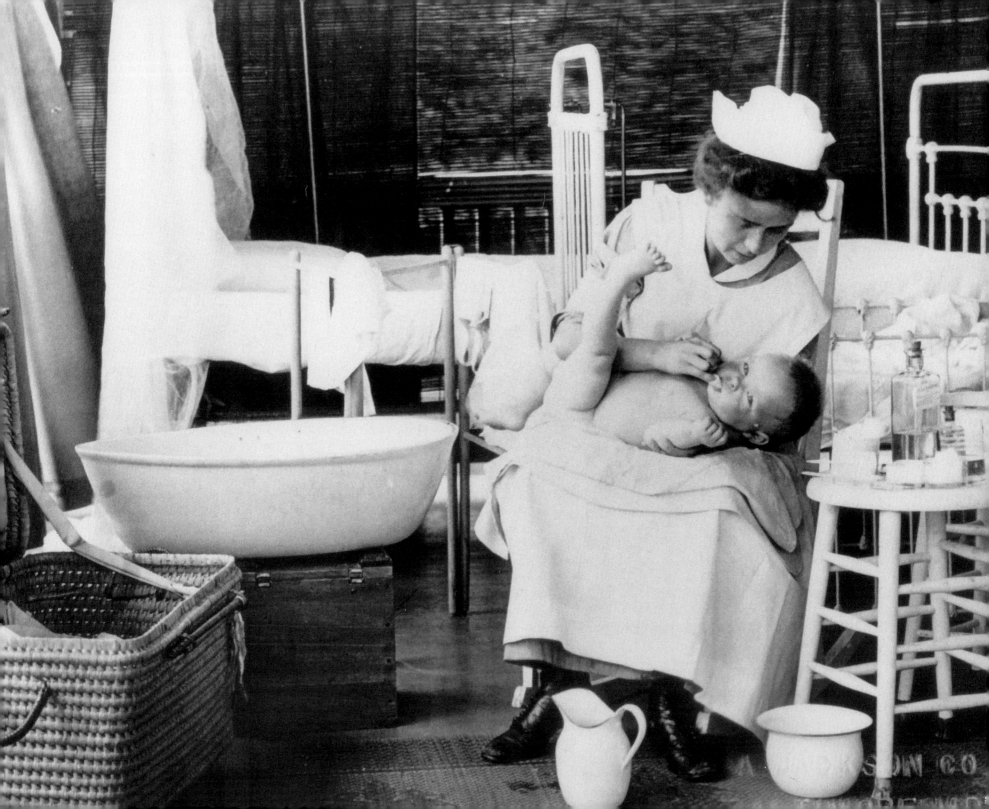

1920

The U.S. population surpasses 100 million.

Congress ratifies the Nineteenth Amendment, which permits American women to vote.

Carrie Chapman Catt forms the League of Women Voters to encourage women's participation in politics.

Prohibition bans alcohol, causing for the next 13 years, an increase in criminal liquor production and sale and the development of the speakeasy.

The League of Nations is formed.

The first radio station, KDKA in Pittsburgh, begins broadcasting with the returns of the Harding-Cox presidential election.

1921

President Harding dedicates the Tomb of the Unknown Soldier in Arlington National Cemetery in Virginia.

The British Parliament grants Southern Ireland dominion status, but six counties in Northern Ireland remain part of the United Kingdom.

1922

Sigma Theta Tau, the national honor society of nursing, is established at Indiana University.

The discovery of insulin revolutionizes medical care for diabetes.

WEAF in New York airs the first commercial, a 10-minute talk by the advertiser that costs $50 but recoups $27,000 in sales.

George Carnarvon and Howard Carter unearth King Tutankhamen's tomb in the Valley of the Kings.

1923

A major earthquake hits the Tokyo area, killing 140,000 people and starting a 39-foot tsunami.

Kodak introduces home movie equipment.

The "Ziegfield Follies" introduces the Charleston to the public.

1924

There are 2.5 million radios in the United States.

1925

In Kentucky, Mary Breckinridge organizes the Frontier Nursing Service, the first rural midwifery service in the United States.

F. Scott Fitzgerald publishes *The Great Gatsby*.

A.A. Milne publishes the first Winnie-the-Pooh book.

Nellie Taylor Ross becomes the first woman to be elected governor of a state (Wyoming).

High-school teacher John T. Scopes is convicted of violating a Tennessee law banning the teaching of any doctrine denying the creation of man as taught by the Bible.

1927

The world's population exceeds 2 billion (doubling the 1804 figure).

The bubonic plague breaks out in Portugal.

Charles Lindbergh makes the first nonstop flight across the Atlantic in the Spirit of St. Louis.

Film industry leaders found the Academy of Motion Picture Arts and Sciences.

1928

Frank Sanborn's company converts its table-model electrocardiograph machine into the first portable version.

General Electric begins the first regular schedule of television programming in the United States.

Kellogg's Rice Krispies cereal snaps, crackles, and pops for the first time.

Walt Disney's Mickey Mouse makes his first appearance in *Steamboat Willie*.

1929

The Wall Street stock market crashes, ushering in the Great Depression.

Alexander Fleming reports his observations on the antibacterial action of penicillium, with the suggestion that the mold culture could be used to inhibit bacteria to help obtain their cultural isolation.

Ernest Hemingway publishes *A Farewell to Arms*.

Werner Forssmann performs, on himself, the first cardiac catheterization with x-ray confirmation.

The Capone gang shoots to death seven members of the rival "Bugs" Moran gang in the St. Valentine's Day Massacre in Chicago.

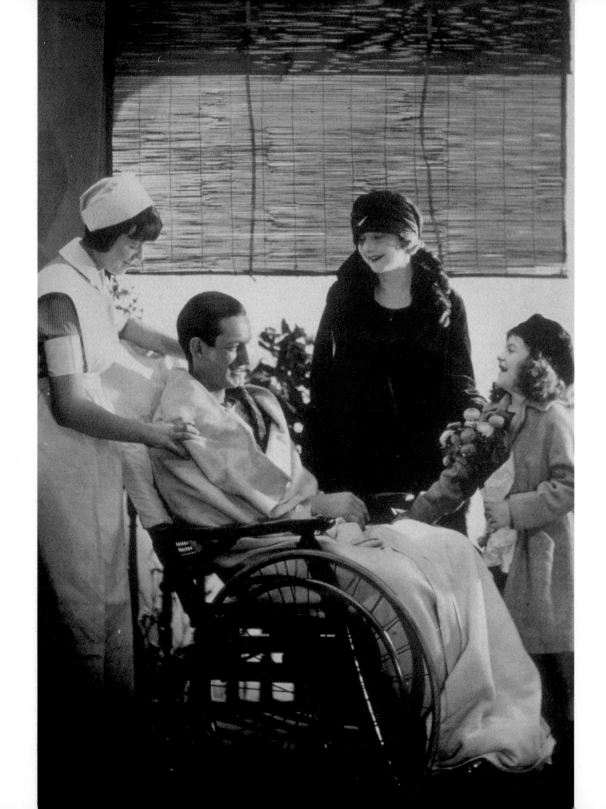

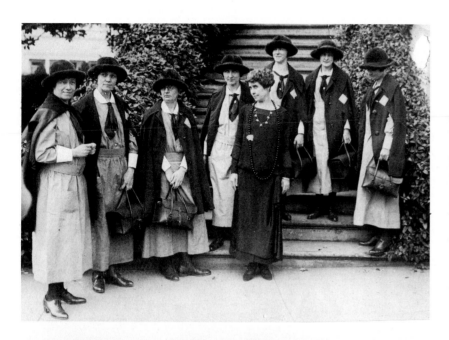

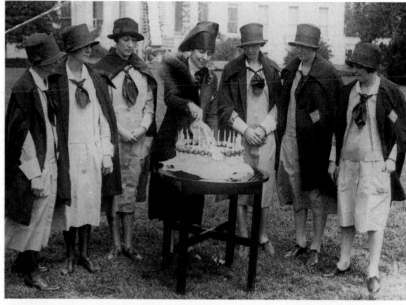

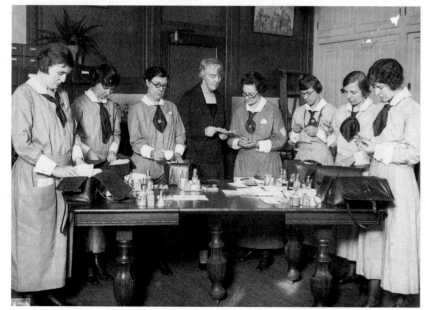

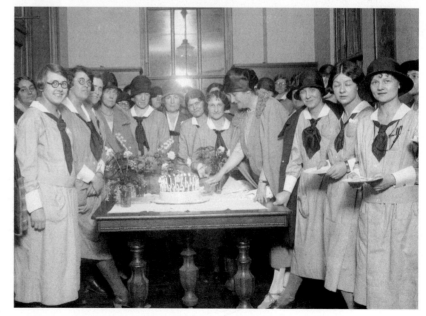

*A*ctivities of the Instructive Visiting Nurse Society (now MedStar Health
Visiting Nurse Association) of Washington, D.C. Mrs. Calvin Coolidge
(top left) was a board member from 1922 to 1928.

24

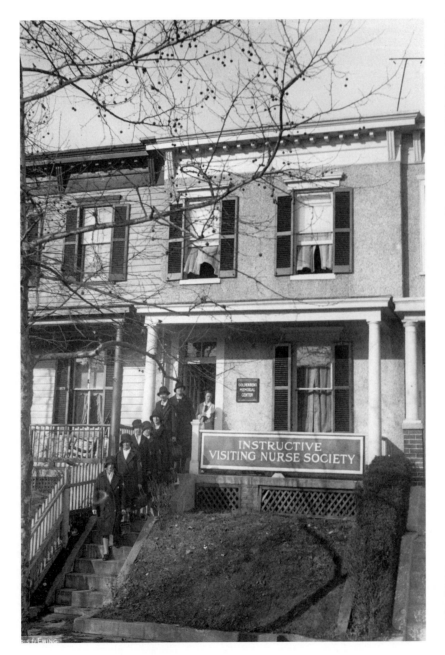

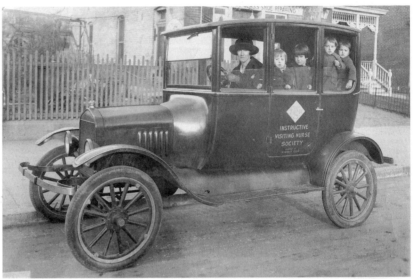

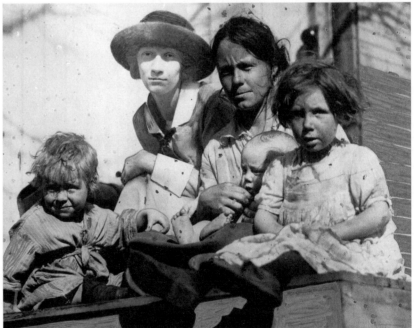

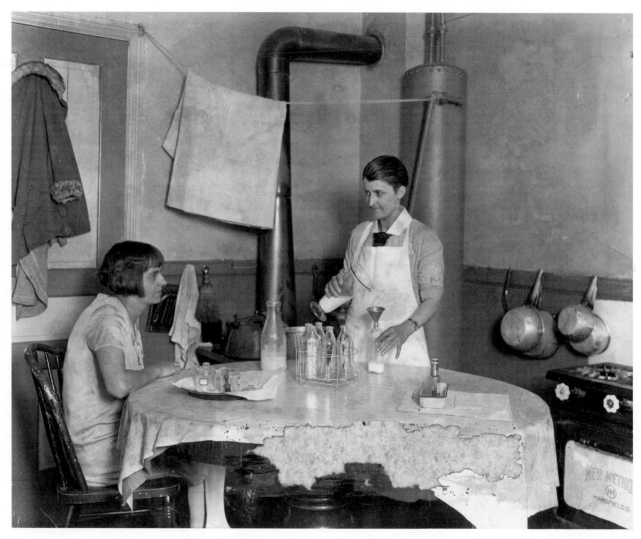

Most of the time, teaching is a one-on-one experience.

I entered the Kentucky Baptist Hospital School of Nursing in June 1925. The nurses' home was on second floor of the hospital and later moved to a house on either Barret Avenue or Vine Street.

On my second day of nursing school, I went to the Operating Room and made supplies for surgery. Classes and lectures began in the fall of 1925. We worked 12 hours a day and had a half day off on Sunday. Our pay was $6 a month.

My most terrible experience was losing a needle of radium while working in x-ray. I didn't know about the loss until I came on duty the next day. The entire x-ray department was in a panic. After looking and looking, I found it in the capsule. Luckily I was not sent home!

Ethel Colcord Mattingly
CLARKSON, KENTUCKY

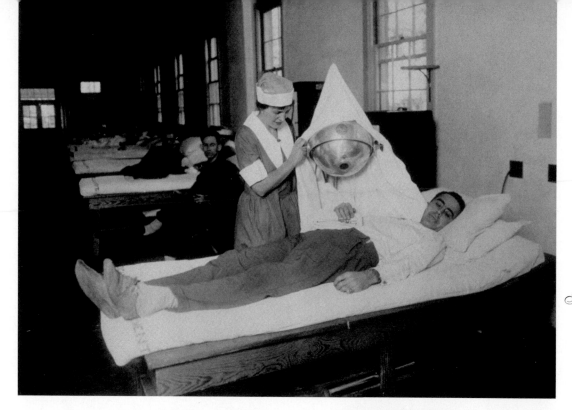

From the early days in hospital nursing, learning to use equipment was an integral part of nursing care.

Top, Before antibiotics, focused light treatments were often used to combat infection.

Bottom, Radiographic equipment.

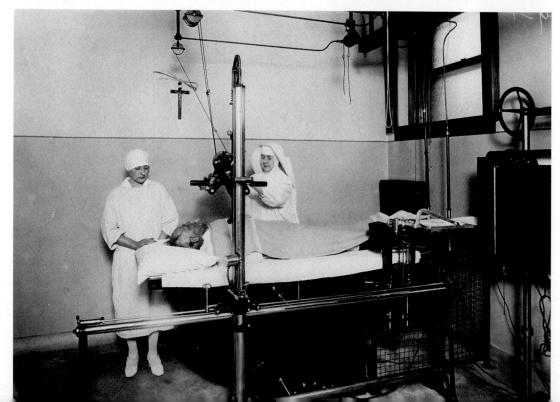

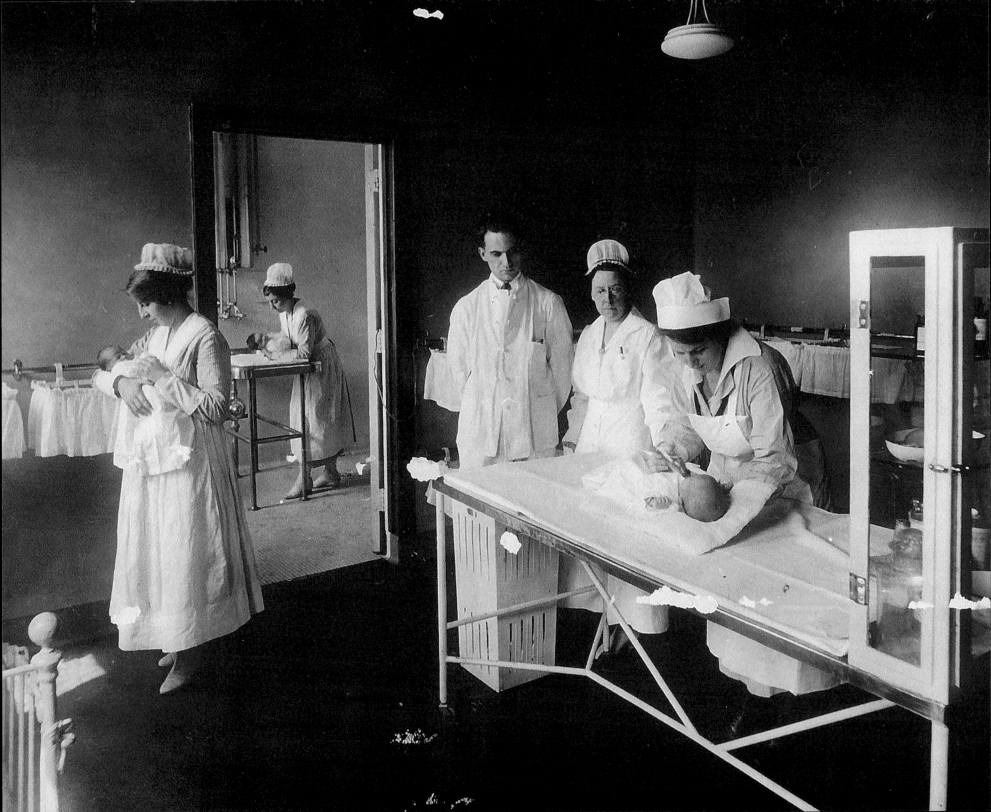

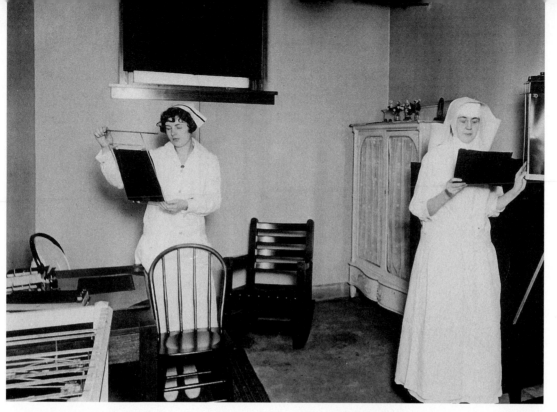

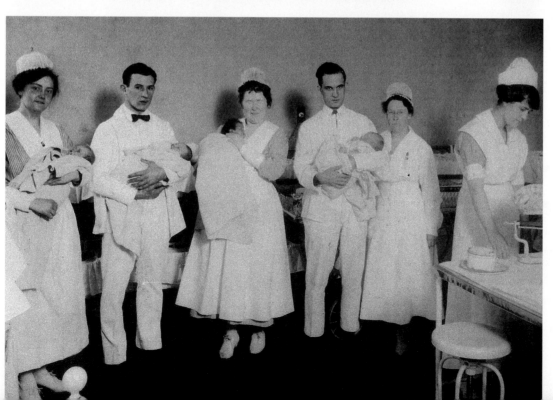

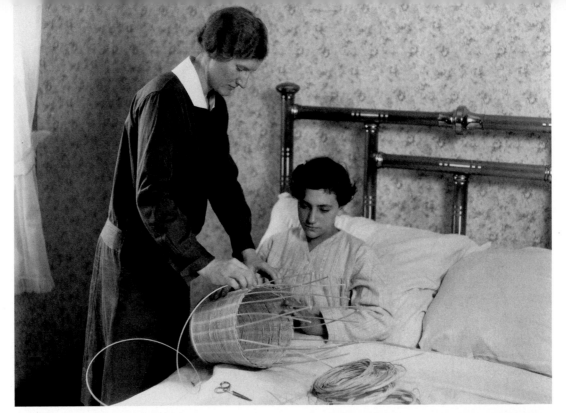

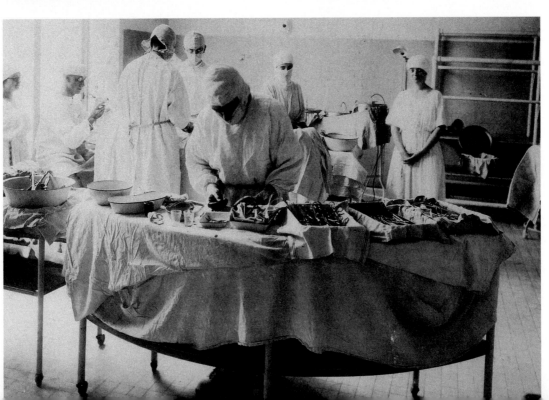

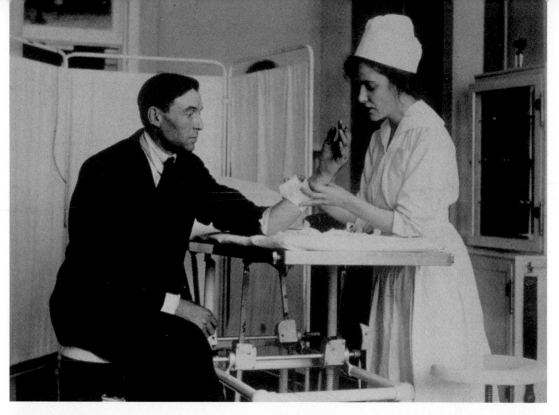

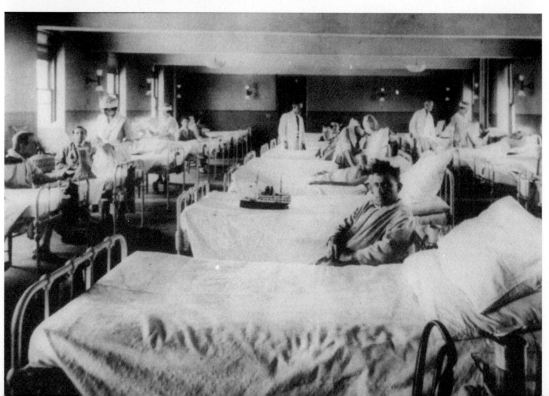

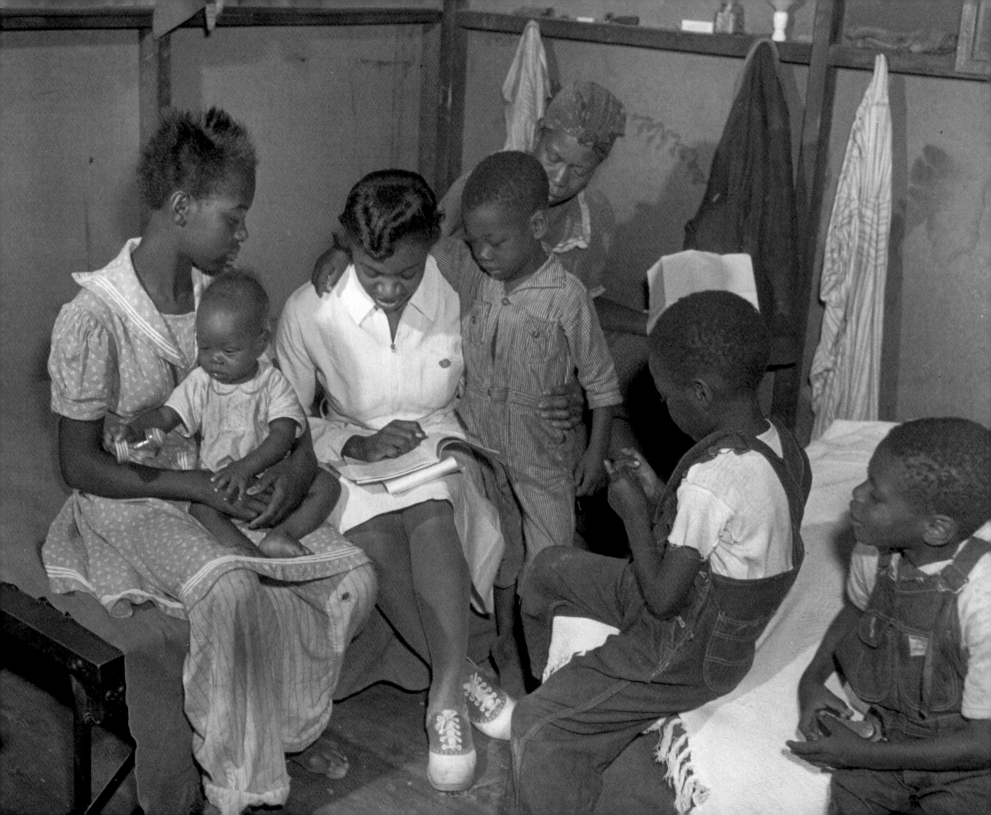

1930

Clyde Tombaugh discovers Pluto, the ninth planet.

Some 4 million workers are unemployed as the Great Depression worsens.

1931

Congress declares Francis Scott Key's "The Star Spangled Banner" the American national anthem.

1932

The Nazi party wins the general elections in Germany.

Wall Street's Dow Jones Industrial Average hits its Depression-era low of 41.22.

A total of 1161 banks fail, nearly 20,000 business go bankrupt, and 21,000 people commit suicide as a result of the Depression.

The worst famine in Russia goes unreported in the Western media.

1933

President Roosevelt uses his "fireside chats" to announce the New Deal: Economic and Social Policy of the United States.

Adolf Hitler comes to power in Germany and proclaims the Third Reich.

Dachau concentration camp is opened, and the persecution of the Jews begins.

Congress repeals Prohibition.

The Association of Collegiate Schools of Nursing (ACSN) is organized to represent schools or departments of nursing associated with universities.

Spam is invented, ushering in a new era of processed foods and additives.

1934

The Dust Bowl hits the United States, devastating farmlands in Kansas, Texas, Colorado, New Mexico, and Oklahoma.

Pavel Cherenkov observes electromagnetic radiation, a discovery of importance for research in nuclear physics.

1935

Gerhard Domagk discovers sulfonamides.

The Social Security Act becomes law, establishing a national old-age pension system.

Reformed alcoholic Bill Wilson anonymously founds Alcoholics Anonymous.

America's first public housing projects are established on New York's Lower East Side.

1936

Soviet leader Joseph Stalin initiates a "great purge" to liquidate his enemies; within 3 years, over 8 million are dead and another 10 million imprisoned.

Approximately 6000 nurses are employed on Works Progress Administration projects.

The British Broadcasting Corporation (BBC) television service commences operation.

1937

The Nazi Third Reich's Hindenburg Zeppelin airship crashes in flames at Lakeland Field, New Jersey.

Amelia Earhart and Frederick Noonan mysteriously disappear over the Pacific Ocean when attempting to fly around the world.

1938

Otto Hahn, Lise Meitner, and Fritz Strassmann split the nucleus of the atom.

Congress passes the Fair Labor Standards Act, providing a minimum wage (25¢ an hour) for the first time.

The broadcast of H.G. Wells' *War of the Worlds* by Orson Welles panics Americans, who believe that Martians are actually invading Earth.

Walt Disney releases the first full-length animated film *Snow White and the Seven Dwarfs*.

1939

World War II begins as German troops invade Poland; France and Great Britain declare war.

Albert Einstein writes a letter to President Roosevelt regarding the possibility of using uranium to initiate a nuclear chain reaction, the fundamental process behind the atomic bomb.

Philip Levine and R.E. Stetson discover the Rh blood group system.

Gone With the Wind premieres in Atlanta.

The National Broadcasting Company (NBC) publicly demonstrates television at the New York World's Fair and announces that it is ready to begin broadcasting for 2 hours a week.

Blood transfusions were a serious treatment requiring a student to sit with the patient while they were given.

Evelyn B. Elder
LOUISVILLE, KENTUCKY

34

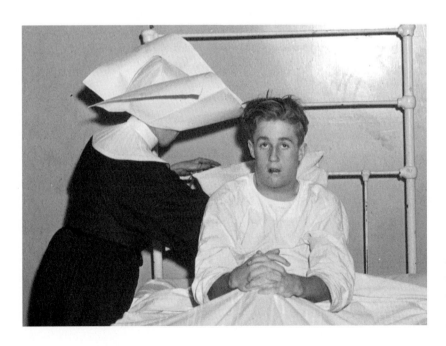

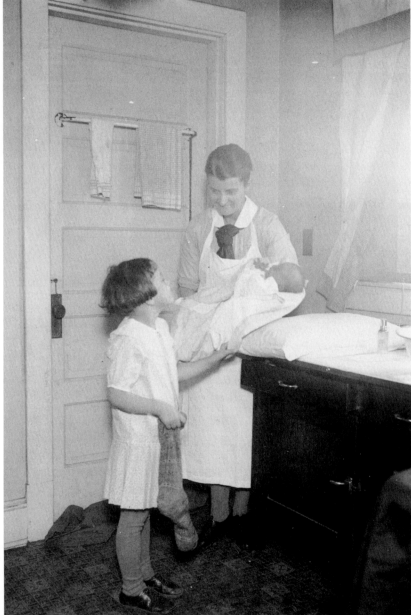

*N*eeded hydration was given rectally by proctoclysis or under the skin by hypodermoclysis. IV infusion came much later.

Katherine Priddy
LOUISVILLE, KENTUCKY

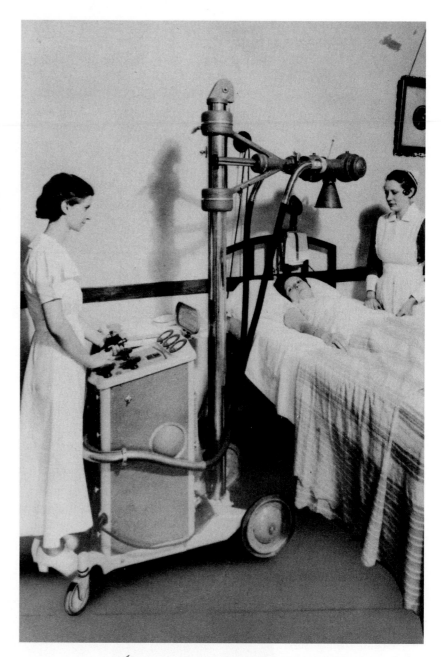

35

A bedside portable x-ray shows the modernization of care.

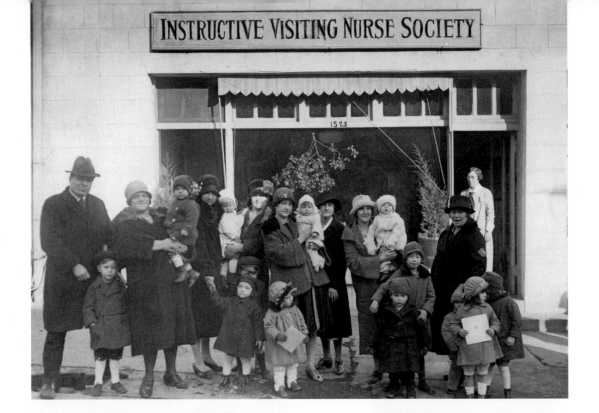

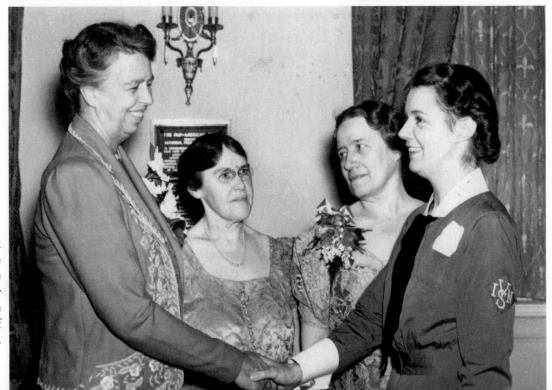

Eleanor Roosevelt meets a nurse from the Instructive Visiting Nurse Society (now MedStar Health Visiting Nurse Association) of Washington D.C.

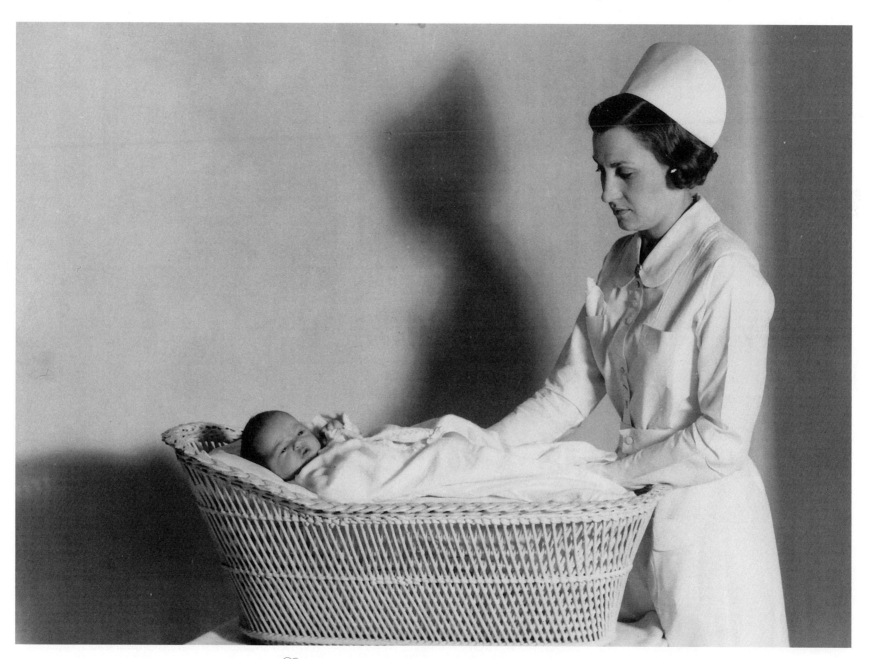

Caring for you in the beginning and throughout your life.

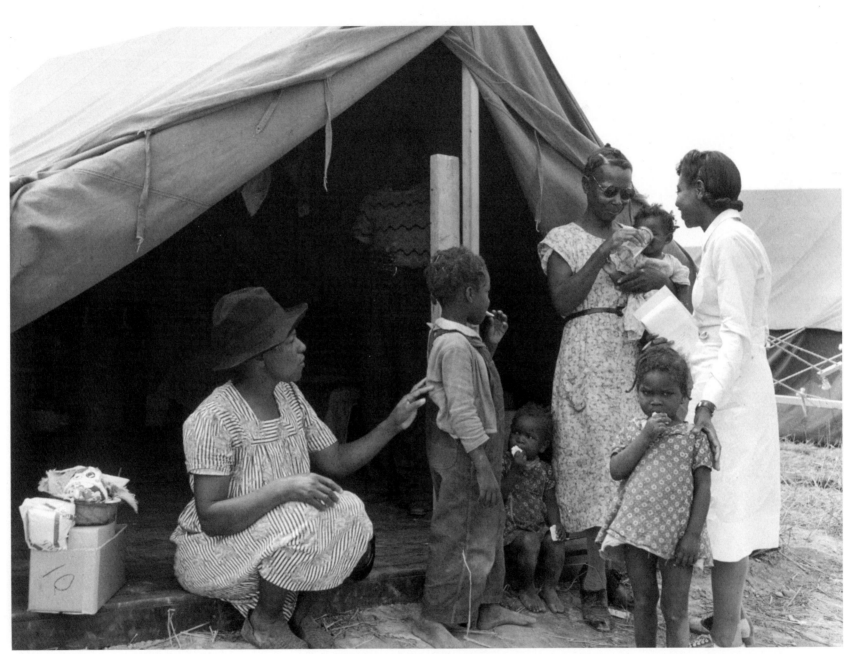

Caring for you wherever you are.

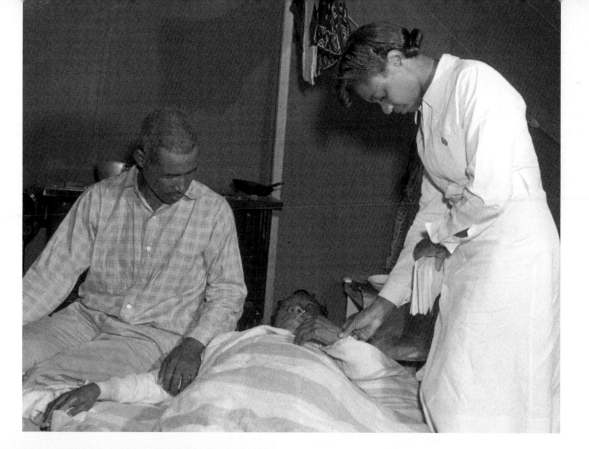

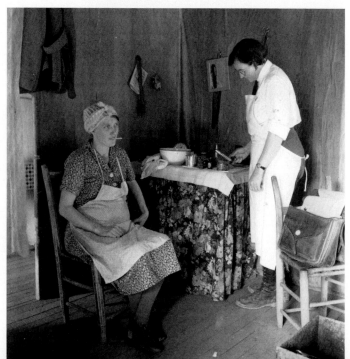

I saw my first miracle when the fever of a pneumonia patient disappeared after he had been given his first treatment of sulfa.

Evelyn B. Elder
LOUISVILLE, KENTUCKY

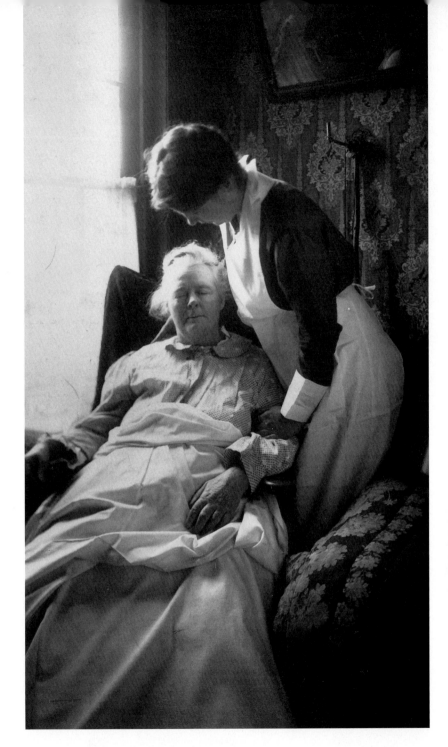

*I*n the 1920s, most RNs worked as private duty nurses in patients' home. The Depression in the 1930s resulted in a sharp decrease in the number of families able to afford private duty nurses, so the opportunities for nurses also decreased dramatically.

The hospitals, always concerned about their alumnae, notified their graduates that they could come back to work as staff nurses. An older nurse told me that after each shift, the nurses would leave through the hospital kitchen. As they walked out, each would pick up a bag of groceries as their pay for that day's work.

Shirley Martin
St. Louis, Missouri

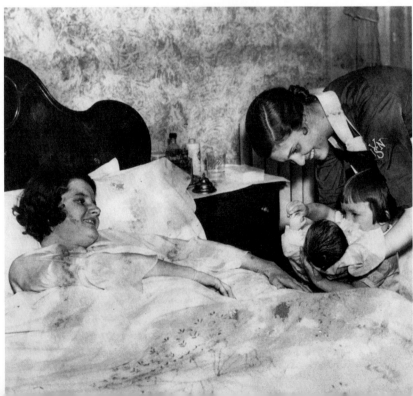

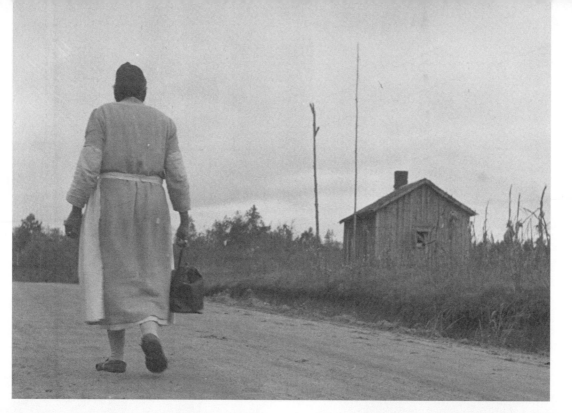

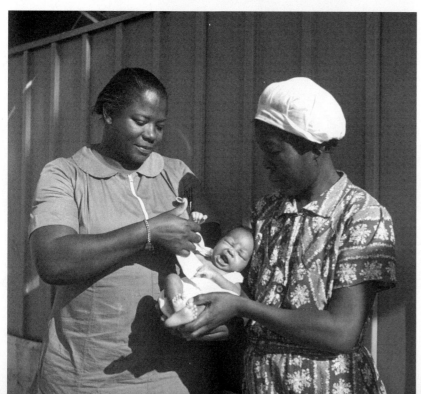

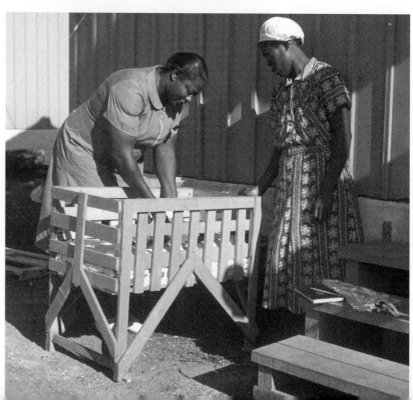

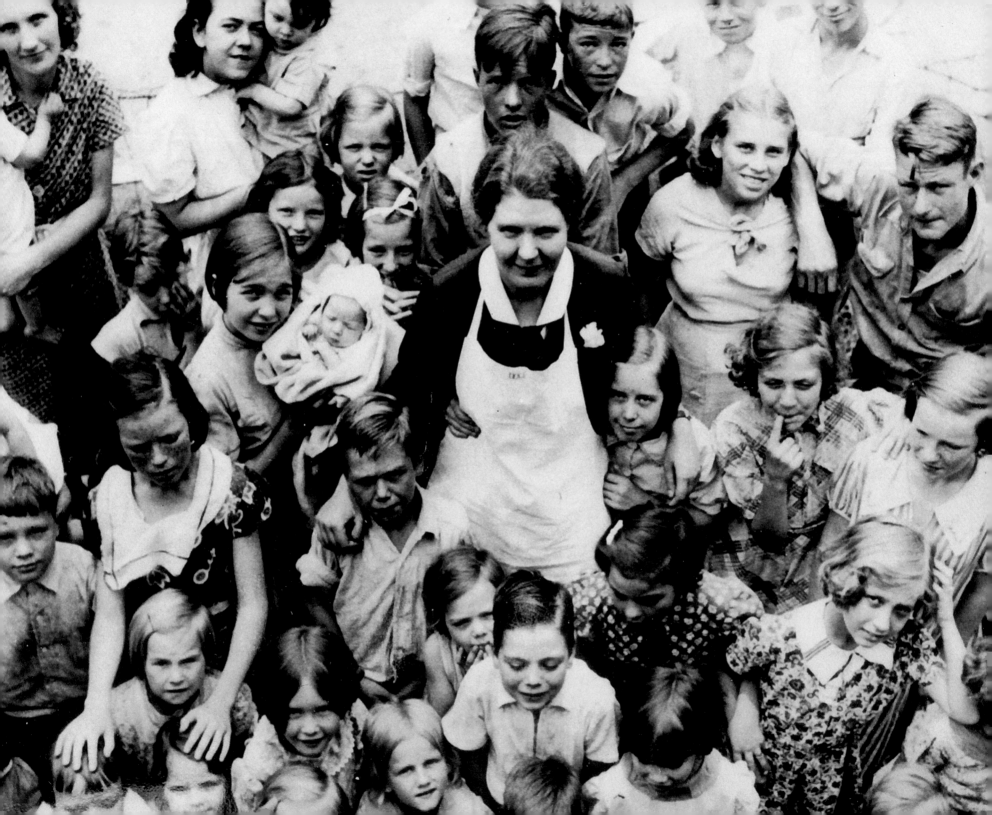

I remember as a young student nurse at Kentucky Baptist Hospital when the 1937 Flood gave my roommate and I our first experience in giving typhoid shots, giving children baths at the corner church. We gave them many baths, in very little water, and we rode down Broadway in a boat with a doctor to help rescue people from the housetops. When a grapefruit truck broke down on Vine Street we carried grapefruit under our uniform aprons (we made many trips) and ate so many to this day grapefruit is my least favorite fruit.

Evelyn B. Elder
LOUISVILLE, KENTUCKY

43

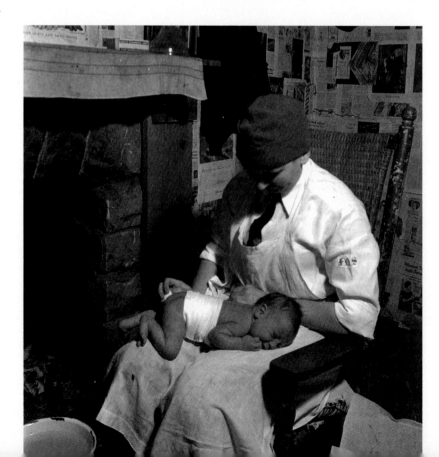

44

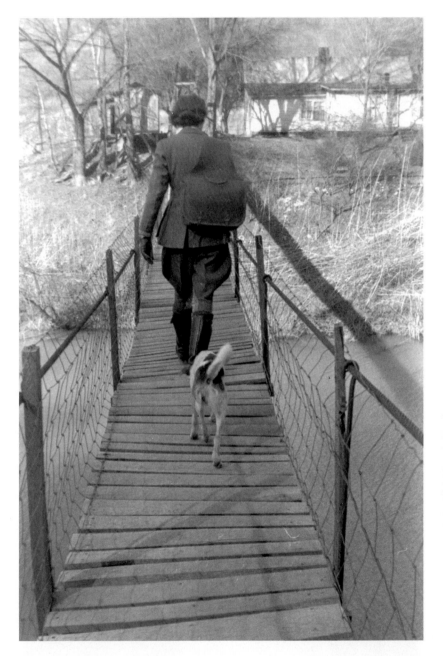

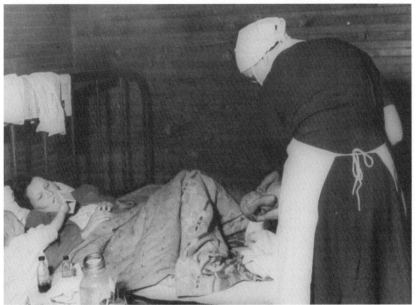

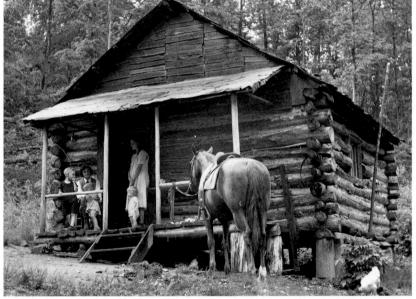

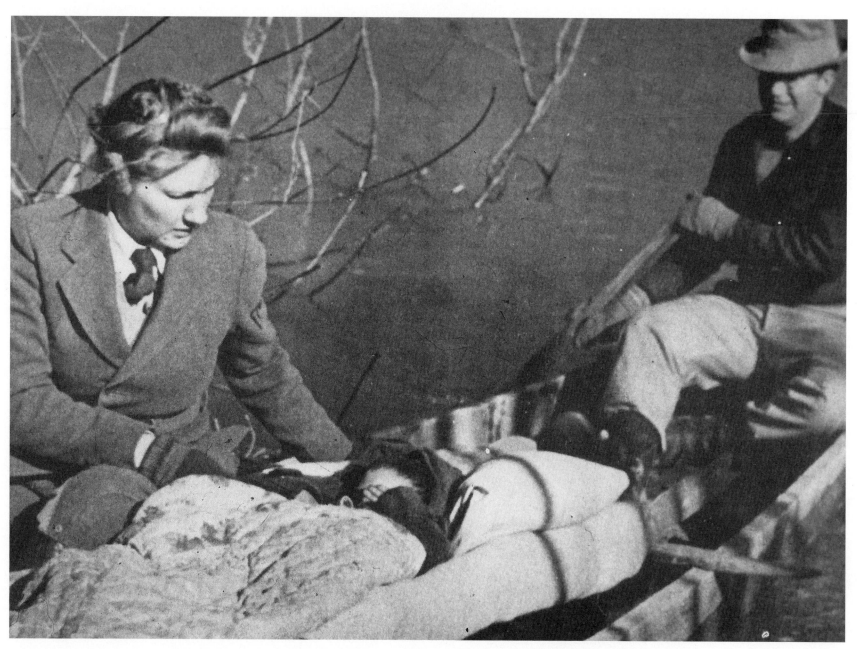

Rural nursing required using innovation and means of transportation that were readily available.

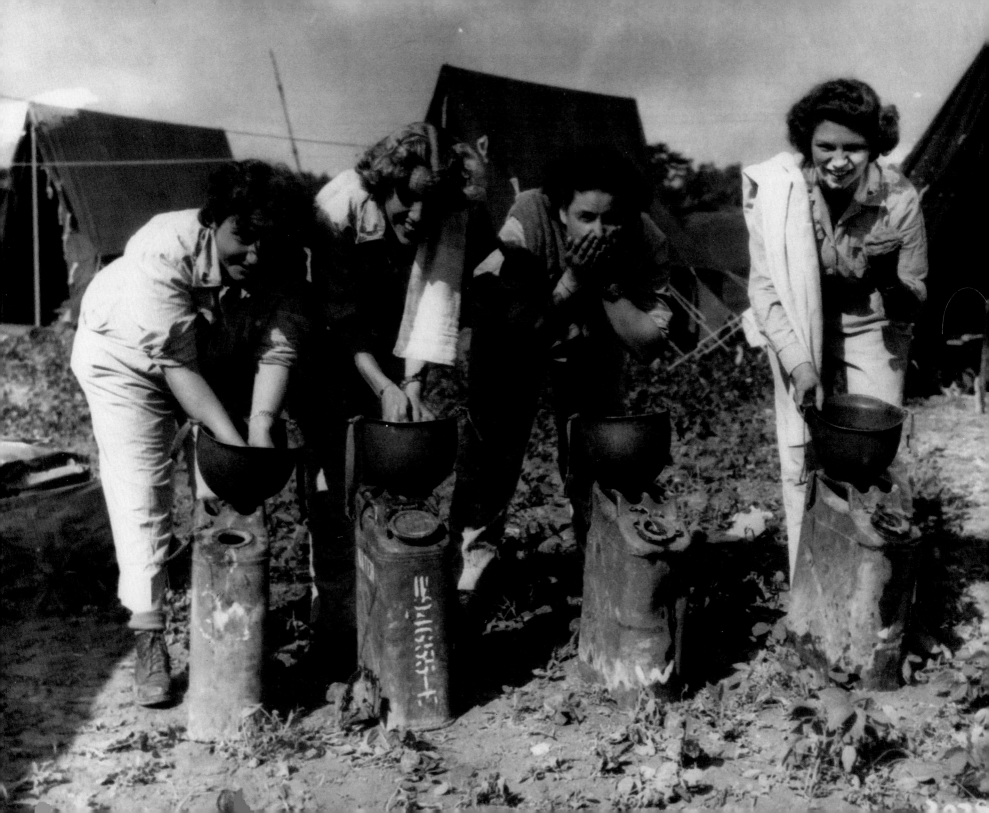

1940

Howard Florey and Ernest Chain develop penicillin as an antibiotic.

Germany invades Denmark, the Netherlands, Belgium, and France and begins a full-scale air war against England.

The National Nursing Council for War Service, representing all nursing groups, is established to serve as a unified group to recruit nurses, providing coordination, information, and communication throughout the war.

African-American surgeon Charles Drew opens American's first blood bank, but segregation rules prevent him from donating his own blood.

1941

The United States enters World War II the day after Japan attacks Pearl Harbor.

The U.S. Treasury issues Liberty Bonds to raise money for the war.

Congress authorizes over $1 million for the fiscal year to assist in the training of nurses for national defense.

1942

Federal appropriations for the training of nurses increase to $3 million.

The Manhattan Project is established to design and build the atomic bomb.

The first Mobile Army Surgical Hospital (M-A-S-H) is introduced but not widely used.

President Roosevelt issues an executive order calling for the internment of 110,000 Japanese Americans.

At the request of the Army, Maxwell House invents instant coffee.

The "Angels of Bataan and Corregidor," Army and Navy nurses, become the only women prisoners in World War II; they spend nearly 3 years in an internment camp, where they care for the sick and dying in the prison hospital.

1943

Congress passes the Nurse Training Act, appropriating $60 million for accelerated, expanded programs in approved schools of nursing. The Act creates the U.S. Cadet Nurse Corps and provides a 36-month basic program, free tuition and fees, free uniforms, and student stipends.

The first class of Army Nurse Corps flight nurses graduates from the School of Air Evacuation at Bowman Field, Kentucky.

Physicians first use the Pap smear to detect cervical cancer; within 20 years, cervical cancer will no longer be the leading cause of death among American women.

Selman Waksman discovers streptomycin, the first antibiotic to be effective in the treatment of tuberculosis.

1944

Nurses in both the Army and Navy are given full military rank for the duration of World War II and 6 months longer.

Allied troops storm the beaches at Normandy under the command of General Dwight D. Eisenhower. Later in the year, France is liberated.

Helen Taussig and Alfred Blalock perform the first subclavian-pulmonary artery anastomosis to correct tetralogy of Fallot, or "blue baby" syndrome.

1945

Penicillin is mass-produced to treat up to 7 million individuals a year.

Allied troops liberate Nazi concentration camps, and the extent of the Holocaust becomes known: almost 6 million dead.

U.S. planes drop atomic bombs on Hiroshima and Nagasaki in August, prompting the Japanese surrender.

World War II ends; total human casualties from the war exceed 50 million.

1946

Winston Churchill coins the term *Iron Curtain* and perceives the beginning of what is to be called the *Cold War*.

The Communicable Disease Center (later the Centers for Disease Control and Prevention [CDC]) opens in Atlanta as part of the U.S. Public Health Service.

Benjamin Spock publishes *The Commonsense Book of Baby and Child Care*, forever changing Americans' thoughts about child rearing.

1947

Full commissioned rank for nurses in the military service is permanently established.

1948

The World Health Organization (WHO) is founded.

1949

President Truman abolishes racial segregation in the U.S. military.

The American Birth Control League, started by nurse Margaret Sanger, becomes Planned Parenthood.

The CIA begins broadcasting to Eastern European areas.

The National Association of Colored Graduate Nurses (NACGN) votes for dissolution, and the American Nurses' Association assumes its responsibilities.

The Volkswagen Beetle enters the market.

47

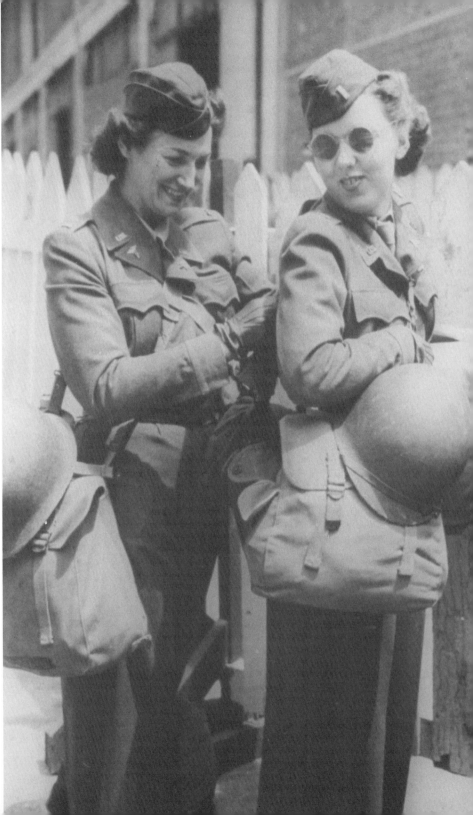

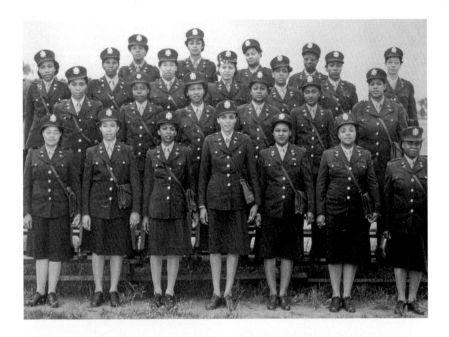

48

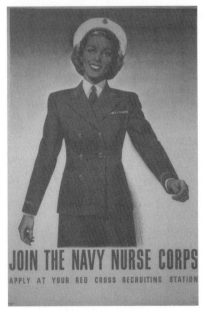

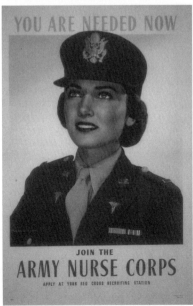

Enrollment quotas were exceeded when 179,000 women joined the U.S. Cadet Nurse Corps.

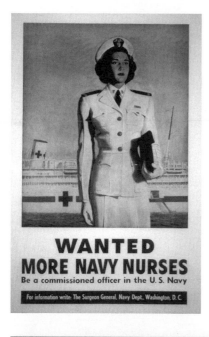

WANTED
MORE NAVY NURSES
Be a commissioned officer in the U. S. Navy

For information write: The Surgeon General, Navy Dept., Washington, D. C.

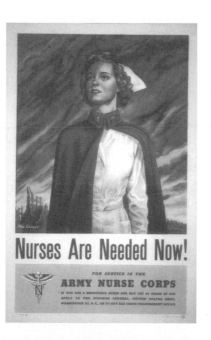

Nurses Are Needed Now!

FOR SERVICE IN THE
ARMY NURSE CORPS

IF YOU ARE A REGISTERED NURSE AND NOT YET 45 YEARS OF AGE APPLY TO THE SURGEON GENERAL, UNITED STATES ARMY, WASHINGTON 25, D. C., OR TO ANY RED CROSS PROCUREMENT OFFICE

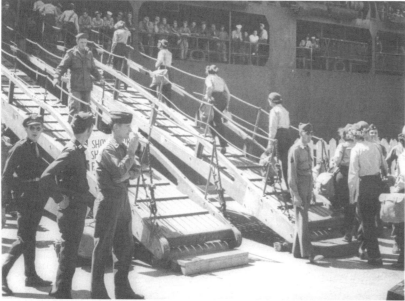

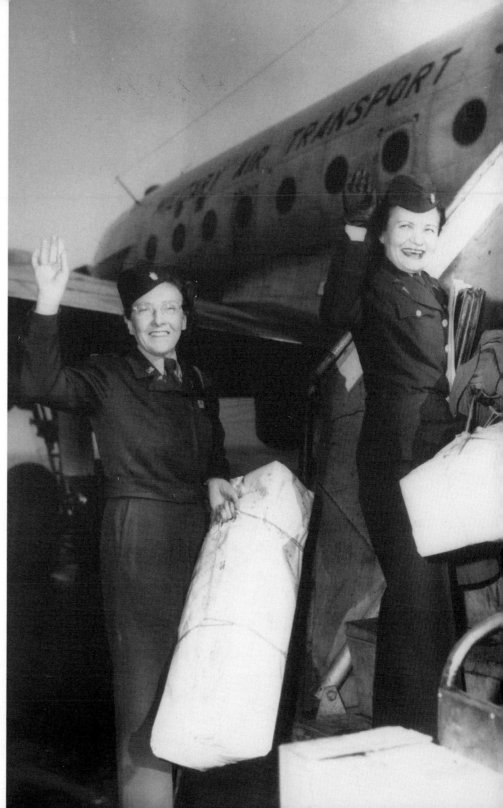

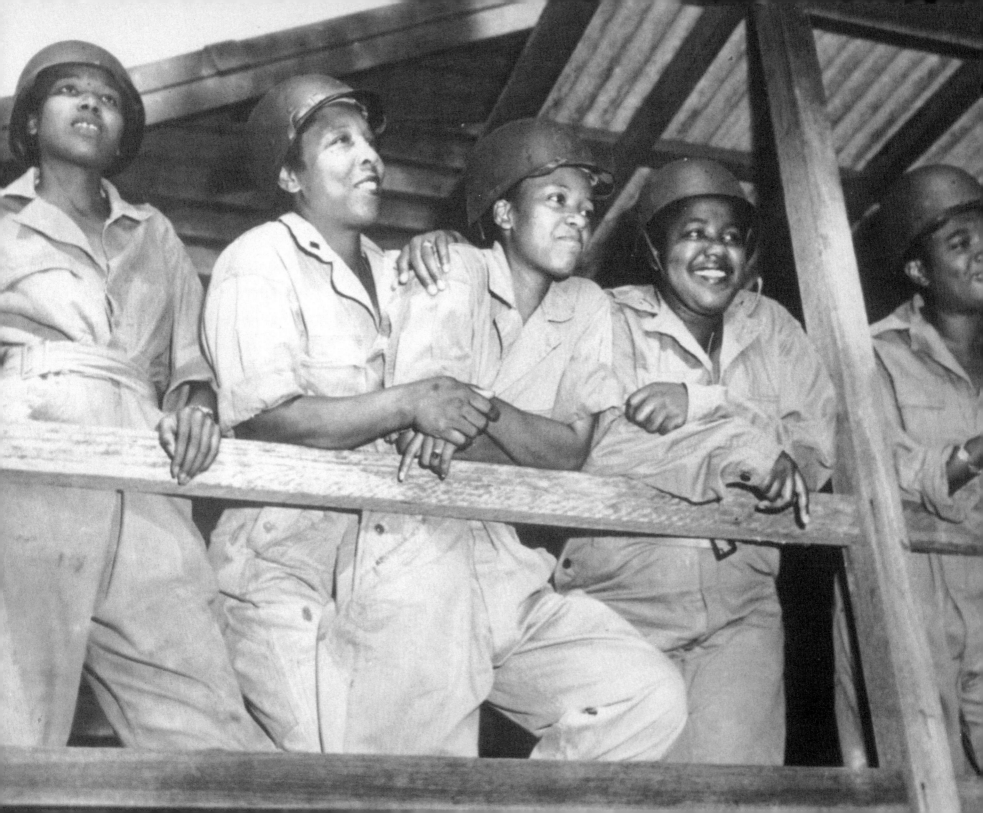

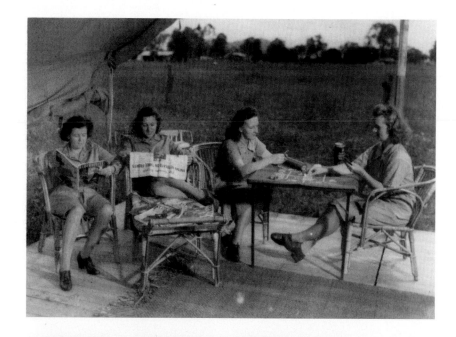

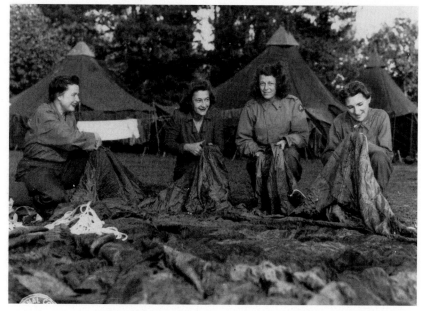

Lunch time at a beach-head hospital in Normandy, a little R&R, and cutting up a German parachute to make scarves.

Following a long ambulance ride from Cairo, Egypt, to Benghazi, Libya, we had our first set-up. Our tents were put over irrigation tanks in a nursery on the outskirts of town. The ward and quarter tents were dug 3 feet into the ground, which made it possible for us to stay in the tents during air raids. One of the doctors, a psychiatrist, was assigned to security, so he routinely made rounds to check for anything suspicious. One day, as he climbed into the command car for rounds, he became alarmed when he noticed a box in the back seat. Convinced the box contained a bomb, he ordered everyone to stay clear of the vehicle. Word of the bomb scare spread quickly, but it was not long before someone who was the wiser stepped forward to tell the good doctor that the contents of the box would do no harm. It was simply the field telephone that was standard equipment in all command cars.

1st Lieutenant Catherine Bane, Honorary Retired USA NC
HOUSTON, TEXAS

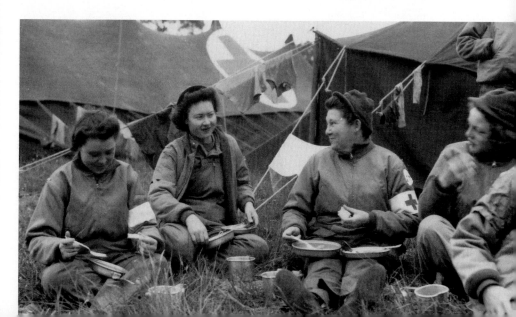

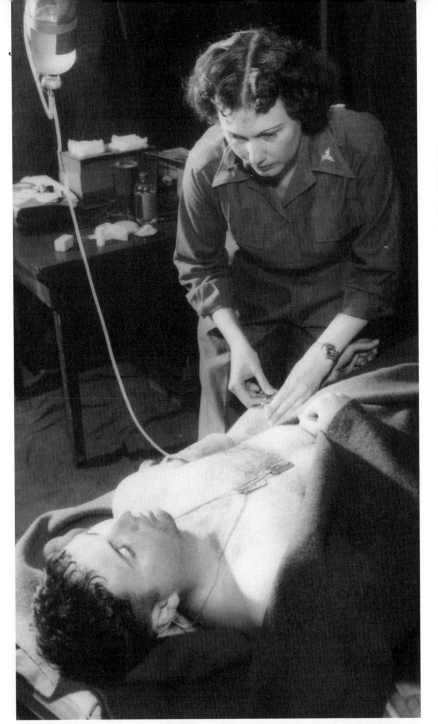

52

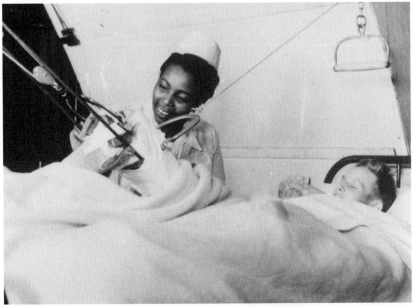

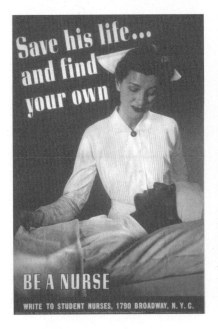

Save his life...
and find
your own

BE A NURSE

WRITE TO STUDENT NURSES, 1790 BROADWAY, N.Y.C.

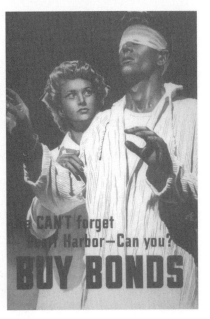

CAN'T forget
Pearl Harbor—Can you?
BUY BONDS

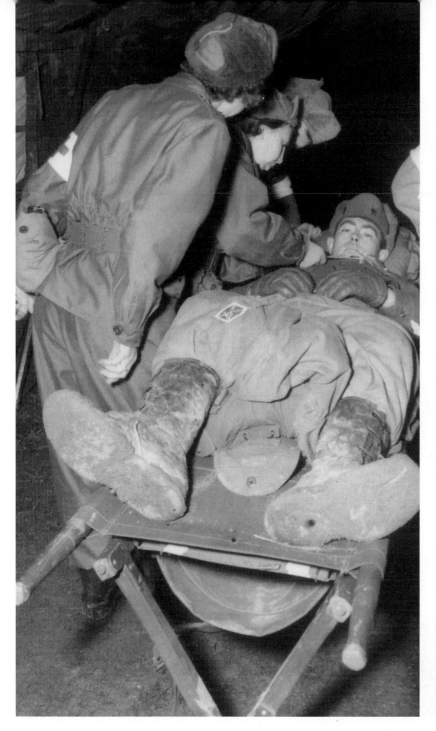

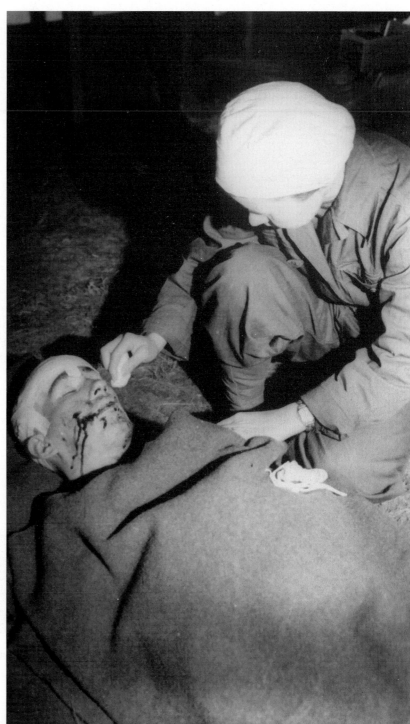

*W*herever needed, nurses were there providing care.

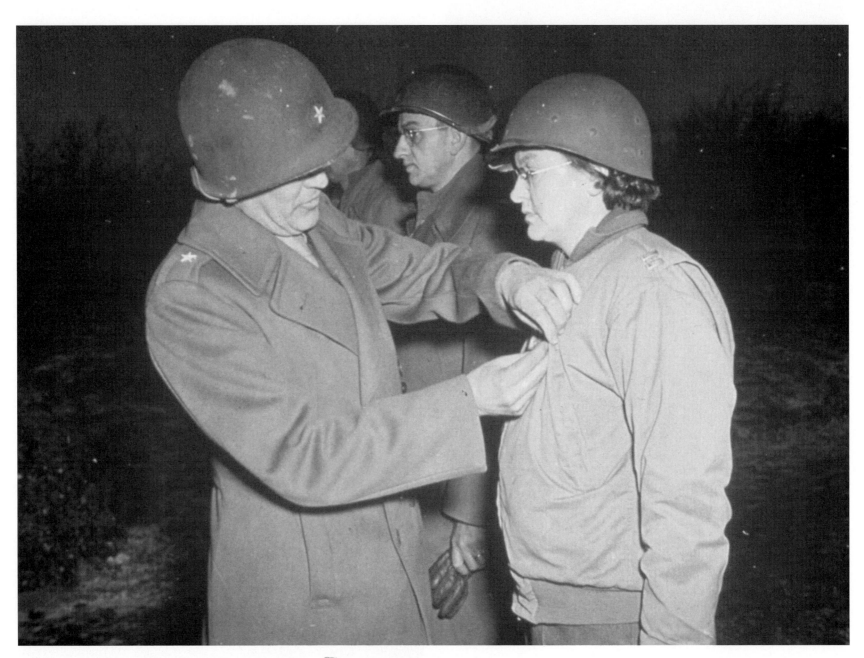

Bravery and service were duly recognized.

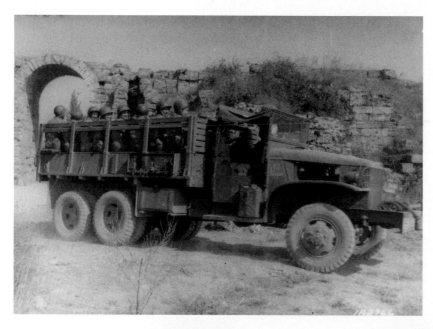

During World War II nurses were stationed in more than 50 countries, providing care in frontline field hospitals, base hospitals, hospital ships, trains, and airplanes.

More than 1600 nurses were decorated for meritorious service and bravery under fire.

A total of 210 nurses died, 16 from enemy action.

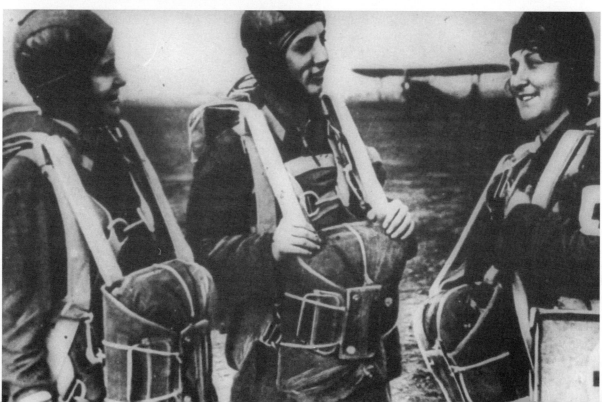

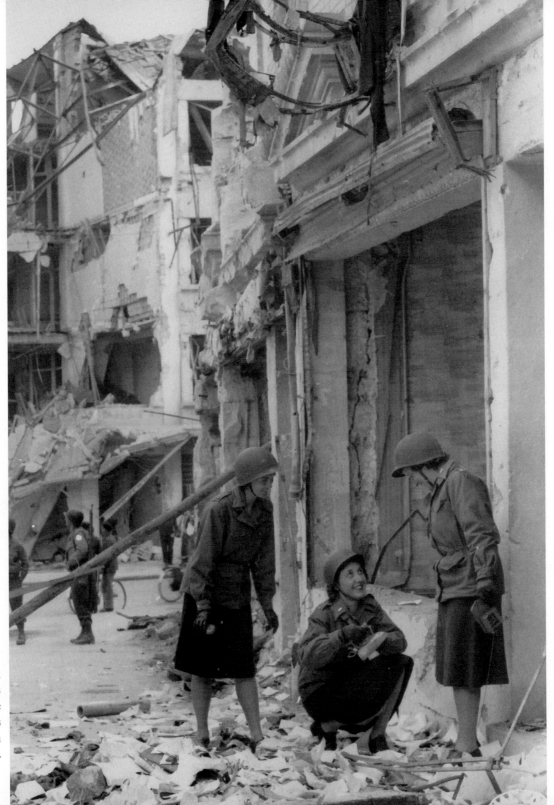

56

Taking a break from duty, these Army nurses find a precious electric iron amid the ruins of a building in Verdun, France.

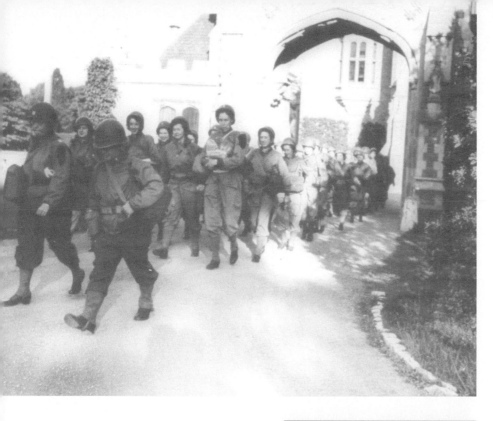

While stationed in Berlin, I spent some time in sick bay over the Christmas holiday with infamous World War II spy, Mildred Gillans, known throughout the world as *Axis Sally*. She was there to have a psychiatric clearance; I had the flu. I noticed that she carried two cans that had once held coffee with her everywhere she went. Curious as I was, I jokingly asked, "What are you carrying around in those cans, gold?" Her response is one I will never forget. She flatly told me that in one can she was carrying a pair of pantyhose for her appearance in court on her treason count and the other was full of cigarette butts. "Now, you don't think the American Red Cross will continue to pass out free cigarettes once I'm in jail, do you?" she asked.

Colonel Betty Ann Beaudry, USA NC Retired
HOUSTON, TEXAS

57

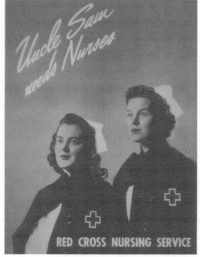

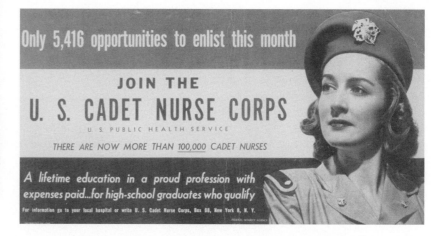

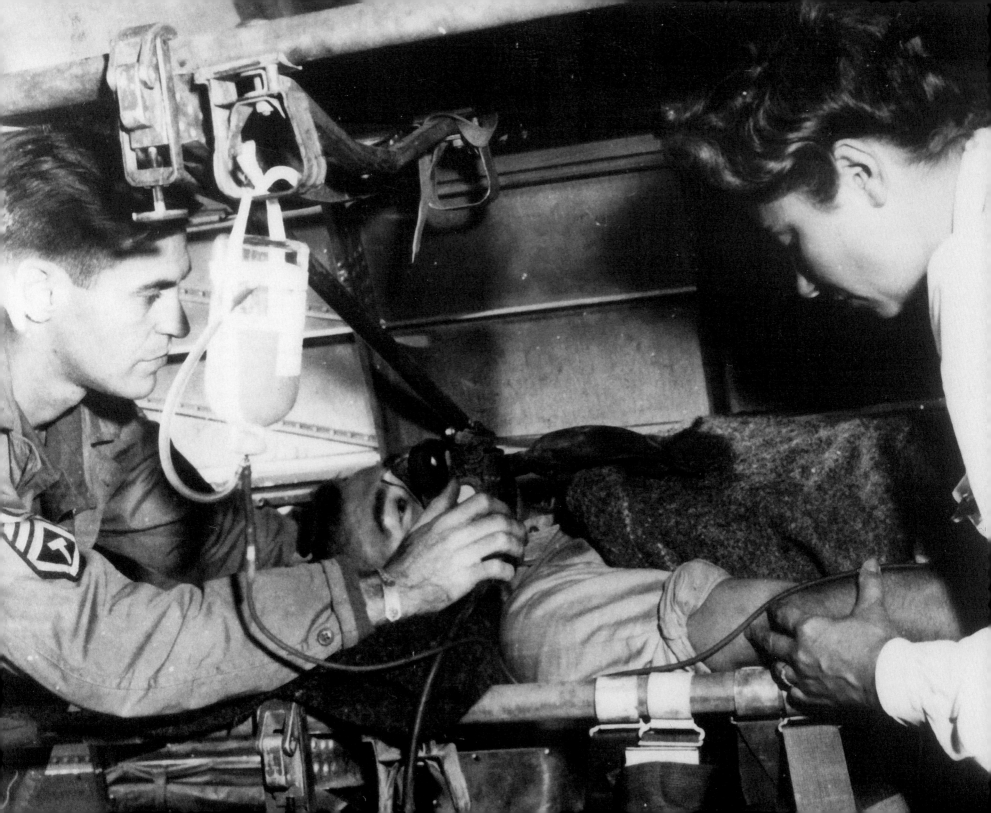

*I*n Libya, we left Benghazi for Bizerte. Our assignment was actually for one platoon to set up in Sardinia and two platoons to set up in Corsica. Our men and supplies would go by boat; myself and five other nurses would travel three at a time by air cargo, a DC-3. When we boarded, we noted the plane's cargo were stacks of boxes marked DYNAMITE. We sat very carefully on the explosives for the short flight across the Mediterranean. The sea below was filled with all kinds of boats headed for Sicily. Our pilot had never been to Sardinia before, and consequently, we landed at the wrong air base. We had to travel across the island by car to get to our platoon but didn't mind as we were so pleased to leave the dynamite behind.

1st Lieutenant Catherine Bane, Honorary Retired USA NC
HOUSTON, TEXAS

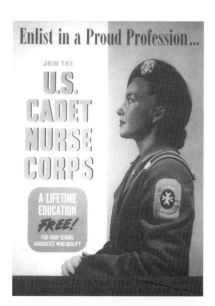

59

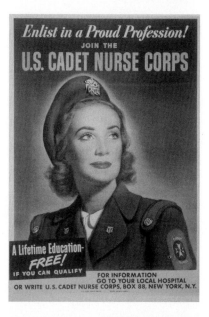

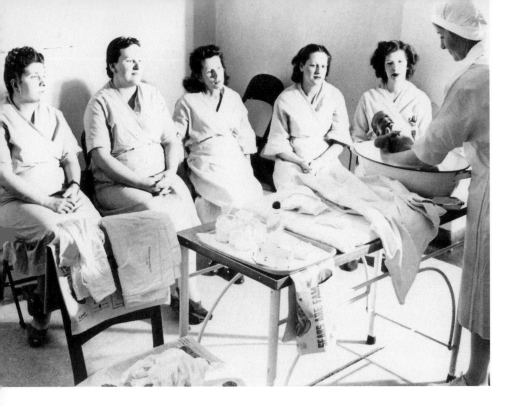

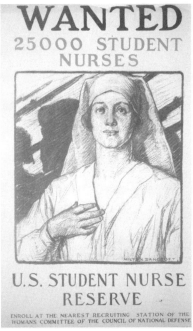

February 22, 1945

*D*ear Kitty,

Here is a letter from your best friend, Shirley, the "probie"! The first 6 months of this program is known as the *Probation Period*, and we are known as *probies*. Right now I am feeling low. I am not certain if I entered a convent, joined the army, was sent to jail, or a combination of all three!

From the first day, we wore the full uniform from morning to night. The collars are so stiff they rubbed my neck raw, and I have a line, like a scar, on both sides of my neck that will be noticeable when I get a tan this summer. Right now we wear the blue checked dress with the collar and cuffs. When we get our caps, we will also begin wearing the bib, and then we will really be dressed up. I suppose we are lucky: we are the first class to wear white hose; the previous classes had to wear terrible black cotton hose during the probation period.

We have classes from 7 in the morning to 4:30 in the afternoon Monday through Friday. We have a 30-minute lunch and 10 minutes between classes. At night, we have compulsory study hours from 8 to 10. Ms. Dawkins, the house mother, makes frequent rounds to make sure everyone is in their room and at their desks. A typical day looks something like this:

5:00 am	Get up	3:00 pm	Anatomy and Physiology class
5:30 am	Breakfast		
6:00 am	Go to chapel	4:00 pm	Anatomy and Physiology lab
7:00 am	Class in Nursing Arts lab		
12:00 pm	Lunch	5:45 pm	Dinner
12:30 pm	To dorm for smoke, bathroom, or whatever	6:00-8:00 pm	Free time in dormitory
		8:00-10:00 pm	Study period
2:00 pm	Chemistry lab	10:30 pm	Lights out

On Saturday we have "housekeeping" duties from 7 in the morning to noon. We are assigned a partner and given assignments to wash and scrub the Chemistry lab and the Diet Therapy lab, dust the books in the library, and dust and polish the faculty offices.

Our classes are Anatomy and Physiology, Chemistry, Microbiology, and Nursing Arts. We have to be in our seat, books open, and not talking when the instructor enters the room. We stand and wait until she reaches the front of the room and tells us to be seated. Nursing Arts is the big class. We spend every morning from 7 to noon in the Nursing Arts lab. This is the room, you will remember, where I took the entrance test, with classroom chairs in front, and then in back are hospital beds, bedside tables and other equipment. We began with the very basic nursing procedures, the bed bath, taking temperature, pulse and respirations, making beds, etc. The reason this class takes so much time is that they are preparing us to go on the "floor." In the first class we were told that on the floor or in the classroom we were always to address each other as Miss ____, and never by our first names. This eventually led to our calling each other by our last names when not in the classroom or on the floor.

The instructor for Nursing Arts is Miss Samples. I have no idea how old she is, but she acts very silly. She has a strong Tennessee accent, so she is difficult to understand. I was told that this is her first teaching job and that she acts silly because she is terribly insecure. Early on she gave a lecture on the care of "fleeres." I had no idea what she was talking about until she demonstrated the placement of flowers in a vase.

Well, so much for the life of a probie. More later.
Shirley

Shirley Martin
St. Louis, Missouri

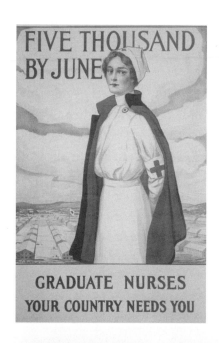

FIVE THOUSAND BY JUNE

GRADUATE NURSES
YOUR COUNTRY NEEDS YOU

61

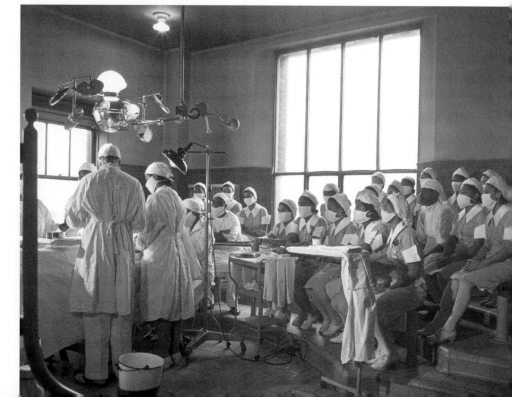

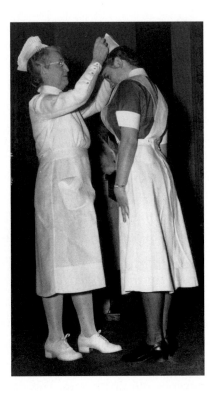

hile we were in nursing school from 1943 to 1946, our uniforms for the first 3 years were black shoes, black hose, blue dress with white collar, cuffs, and white apron. Then we got a white bib and a white cap. In our senior year, we got a narrow black band on each of our caps.

We worked hard but we had fun. We had hands-on learning.

Lena Hurst
LOUISVILLE, KENTUCKY

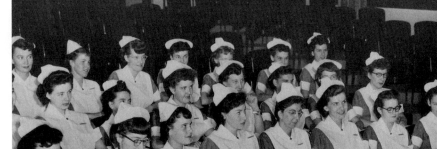

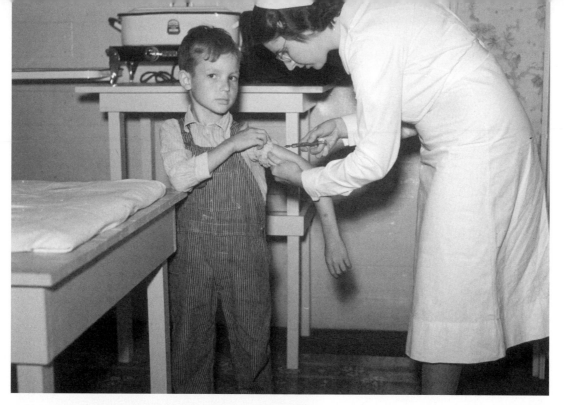

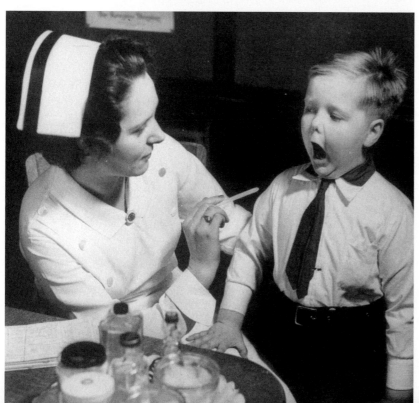

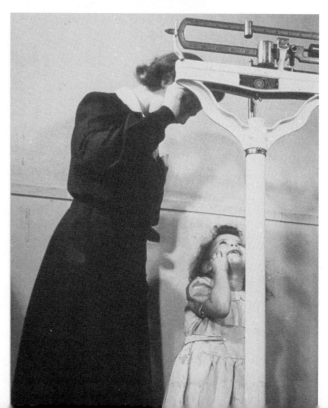

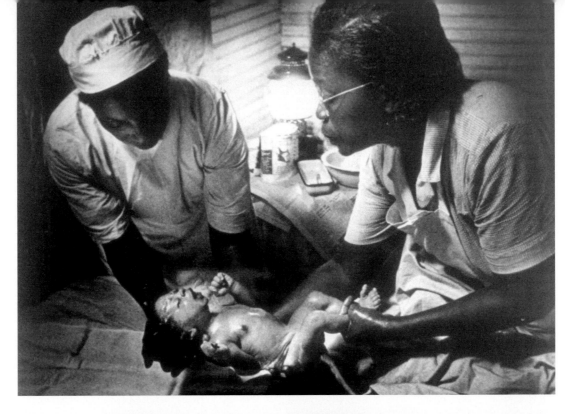

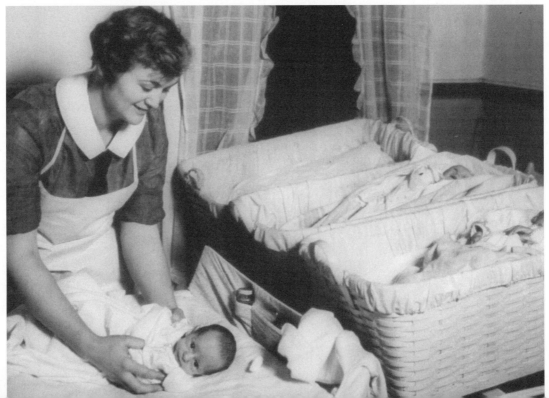

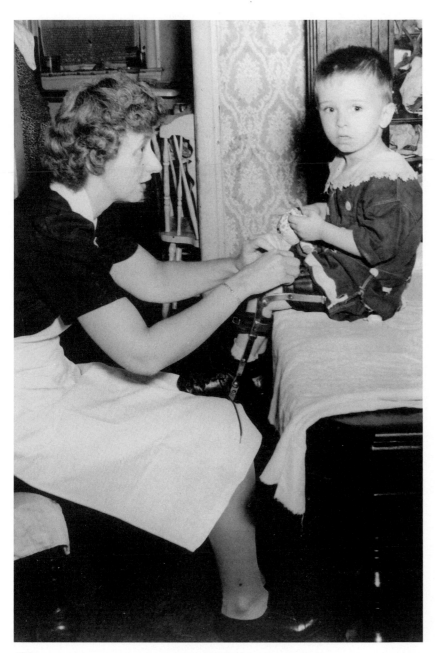

*P*olio became an all too frequent challenge for nurses.

*M*ethods of healing and administering to the sick have made great strides. I remember a youngster on the crippled children's ward whose osteo-infected leg was being treated with maggots inside his cast, to cleanse his wound. When the maggots had eaten their "fill," they crawled out the window of his cast, leaving a screaming little scrapper and a terrified student nurse. The maggots were captured and sent to be incinerated so as not to spread more infection.

Hot turpentine strips were the order of the day for treating an acutely infected distended abdomen.

Despite the lack of modern methods, medicine, and "machinery," critically ill patients were able to walk or be wheeled out of the hospital–made well with kindness, prayers, and TLC.

Katherine Pirdy
Louisville, Kentucky

65

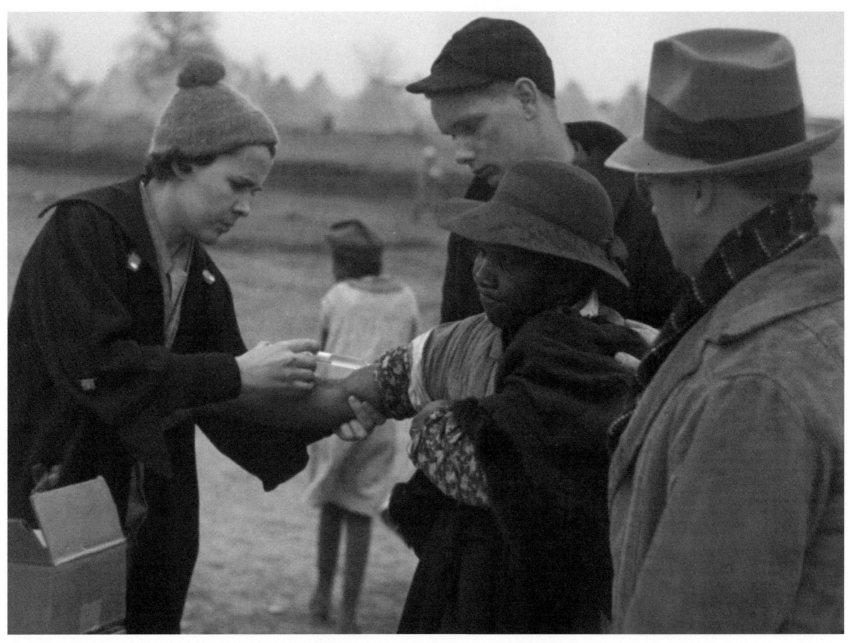

To help stop the spread of infectious diseases, nurses went into communities to provide immunizations to rural farm and migrant workers.

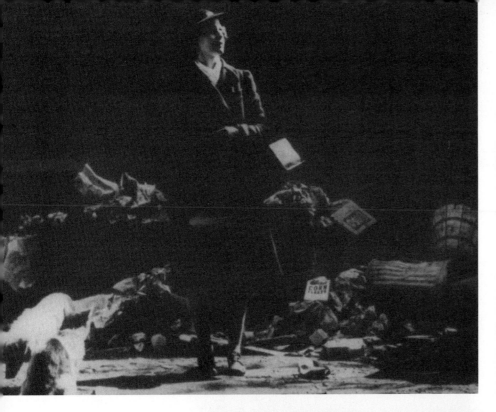

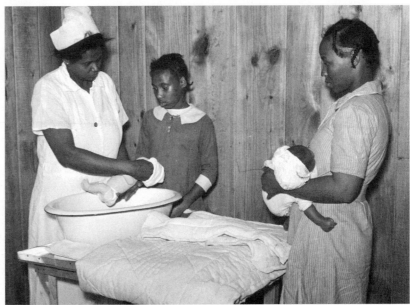

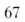

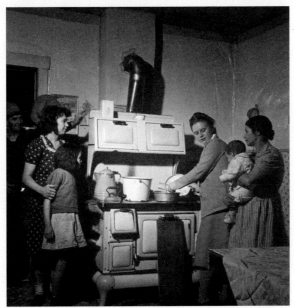

A nutrition lesson centers around greens and canned vegetables.

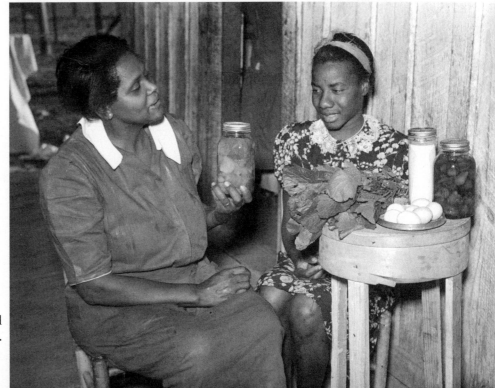

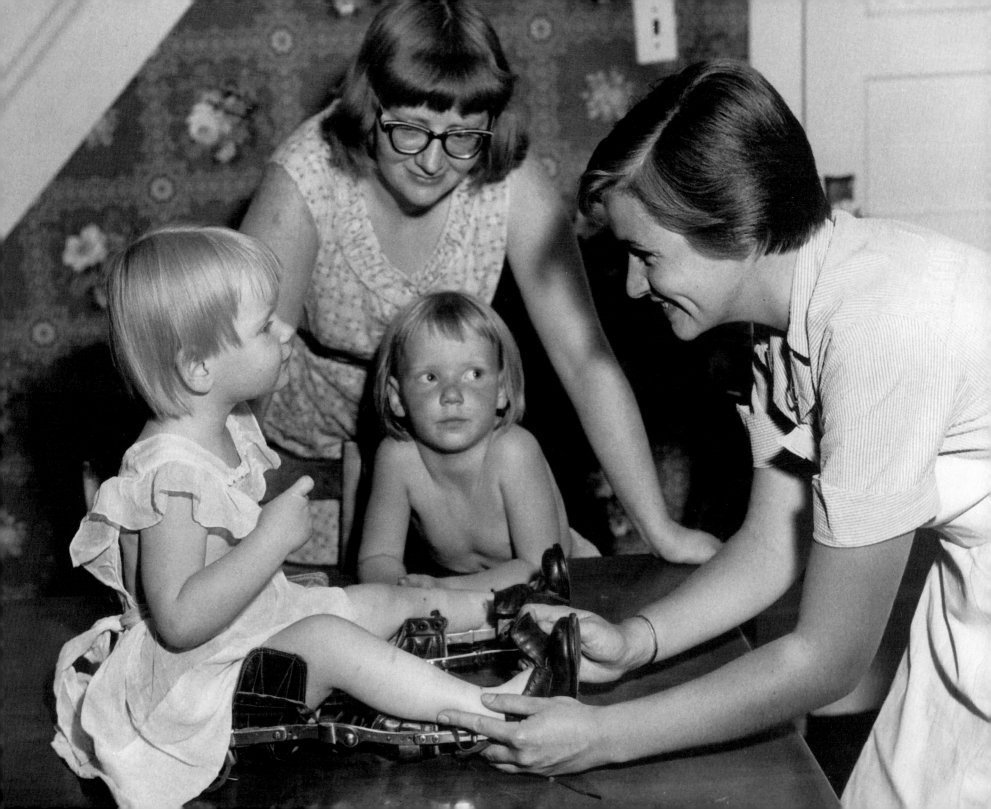

1950

American musicians, including Ira Gershwin and Louis Armstrong, dominate popular music.

Polio is a major public health problem affecting over 50,000 Americans.

Snoopy, Charlie Brown, and the rest of the Peanuts gang premiere in Charles Schulz' comic strip.

North Korea invades South Korea, sparking the Korean War.

Senator Joseph McCarthy begins his anti-Communist witch hunt.

President Truman sends U.S. military troops as part of a United Nations effort in the Korean conflict.

M-A-S-H units are actively used to treat the wounded close to the battle area in the Korean War. These "portable" hospitals significantly decrease a soldier's time from injury to surgical treatment.

1951

I Love Lucy with Lucille Ball and husband Desi Arnaz begins its 6-year run.

The American Nurses' Association, the National Foundation of Infantile Paralysis, and the American Red Cross found a volunteer, mobile, polio nurse specialty group that serves in communities during polio epidemics.

John Gibbon, Jr., creates the first heart-lung machine.

1952

The first successful open heart surgery is performed at the University of Minnesota.

Associate-degree nursing programs are piloted in seven strategically positioned community colleges.

1953

Dr. Virginia Apgar publishes her neonatal scoring system known as the *Apgar score*.

James Watson and Francis Crick determine the double-helical structure of DNA.

Elizabeth is crowned queen of the United Kingdom of Great Britain and Northern Ireland.

Experiments in mice link cancer to tobacco tar.

Commercial advertising expands now that 20 million households have television sets.

1954

French colonial rule in Vietnam weakens when Viet Minh rebels take Dien Bien Phy, resulting in the division of Vietnam into northern and southern regions.

In *Brown v. Board of Education of Topeka, Kansas*, the Supreme Court rules unanimously that racial segregation violates the Fourteenth Amendment.

1955

The American Nurses Foundation is founded to conduct research, provide research grants, and publish scientific work.

Male nurses are commissioned in the Army Reserve for assignment to Army Nursing Corps.

Jonas Salk's killed-virus polio vaccine is released for use in the United States.

Rosa Parks refuses to go to the back of the public bus and is arrested in Montgomery, Alabama, precipitating the bus boycott that ignited the Civil Rights Movement.

"Rock Around the Clock" and "Maybelline" hit the popular music charts.

1956

Ray Kroc purchases a hamburger franchise from the McDonald brothers and erects the first "Golden Arch."

Prince Rainier of Monaco marries actress Grace Kelly.

Elvis Presley tops the charts with "Love Me Tender," "Hound Dog," and "Heartbreak Hotel."

1957

The Soviet Union launches Sputnik I and II into space orbit, triggering the space race.

Albert Sabin develops the live-virus polio vaccine.

When nine African-American students attend all-white Central High School in Little Rock, governor Orval Faubus calls out the Arkansas National Guard to "prevent violence" by blocking their access, prompting President Eisenhower to mobilize the Army to escort the students into the school.

ABC reluctantly airs Dick Clark's "American Bandstand" nationally.

Dr. Seuss publishes The Cat in the Hat.

1958

The National Aeronautics and Space Administration (NASA) is established.

American Express debuts the credit card.

1959

Fidel Castro becomes premier of Cuba, and the Cuban Revolution begins.

Alaska and Hawaii become the forty-ninth and fiftieth states to join the Union.

Edmund Hilary and Tenzing Norgay become the first humans to reach the summit of Mount Everest.

An armistice is signed at Panmunjom, South Korea, to end the Korean War; human casualties in the war reach 1.9 million.

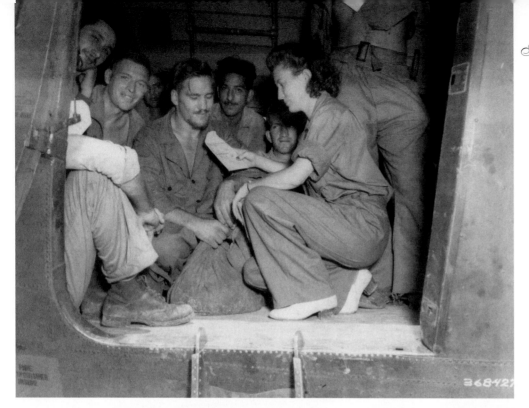

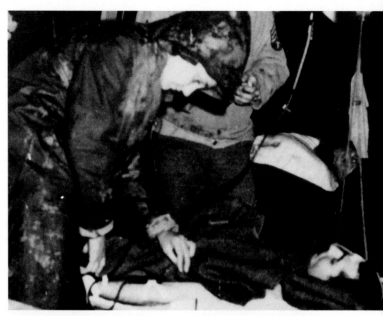

The Korean War again took nurses to M-A-S-H units and other hospitals close to the battlefields.

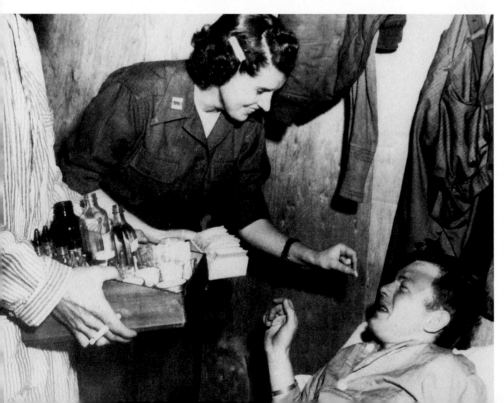

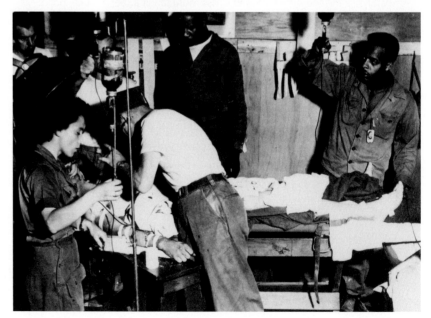

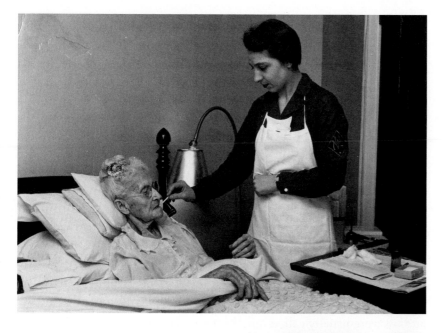

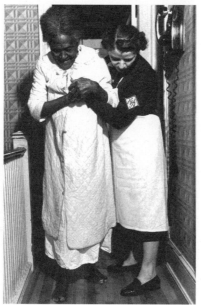

My most powerful memory of nursing is when as a new probationer, I had to give my first "shot." This was in a hospital-affiliated school of nursing in the early 1950s. We were exploited as a labor force, and schooling was sandwiched in off hours. We had been taught how to give a shot in the lab, but this was to be done on a real, live person. I was 17 and afraid of harming her.

She seemed barely alive to me. She was a tiny-waisted, 85-pound, pale, gray-haired grandmother. Her buttocks resembled a well-used pincushion. They were lumpy with fluid and scarred with red puncture marks and orangish blue splotches. Her ischial tuberosities protruded, and her sad-looking skin sagged. She required hot soaks to these painful areas. She whimpered when it came time for her every-4-hour, round-the-clock injections of penicillin and streptomycin in oil suspension. It was not only the fact that 5 cc of each required two separate syringes, but the oil suspension obliged a slow, painful time for release from the syringe and its necessarily large-gauge needle.

My first attempt ended with both of us crying. I sobbed to the head nurse that she would have to do it because I just couldn't. She patiently sat me down and explained that I needed an attitude adjustment. The patient had subacute bacterial endocarditis, and she would definitely die without the antibiotics. She went on to say that when she started nursing, she had seen many die from this disease. Before the discovery of antibiotics, death was almost certain.

By the time I left her desk, I realized that even though giving the shot seemed so painful to both of us, it was really a blessing. I always think of this whenever I have to give any shot. It has made me look beyond the momentary pain to the eventual effect.

Joan Kasson
COLUMBUS, OHIO

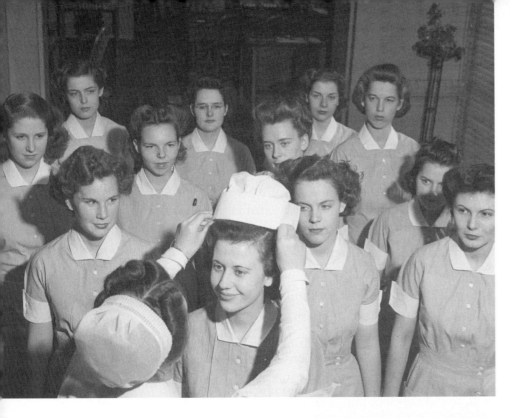

Our small class entered nurses' training in January 1951. We were given rooms in the old house next to the hospital. Miss Ollie Wilkerson looked after and encouraged us. We were her "little girls."

Starting in May 1951, the students ran the hospital from 3 pm until 7 am. Our class would attend classes in the morning and then work either 3 pm until 11 pm or 11 pm until 7 am. My first day on duty my patient died. That was a terrible experience.

Before I had a class in operating room technique, I was sent to O.R. and scrubbed on my first major case. I didn't know one instrument from another. The anesthesiologist, Dr. Fred Williams, was able to come to the table and show me what instrument the surgeon was asking for. We were on call for surgery every other night, and we were usually called out. At the end of my 8-week rotation, I had scrubbed on 175 major cases. Needless to say, I knew where I wanted to work when I graduated.

Juanita Mattingly Wagner
ANCHORAGE, KENTUCKY

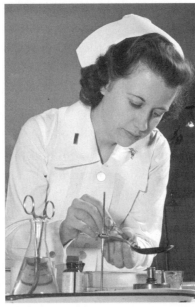

Sometimes, preparing medication for injection first meant melting the substance in a large spoon over an open flame and then drawing it into a syringe for administration.

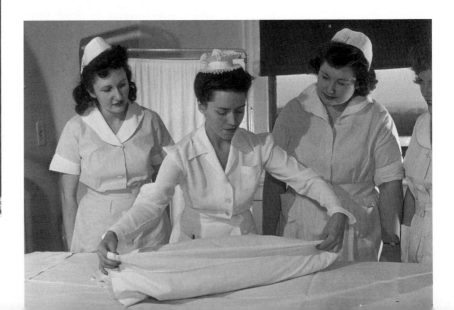

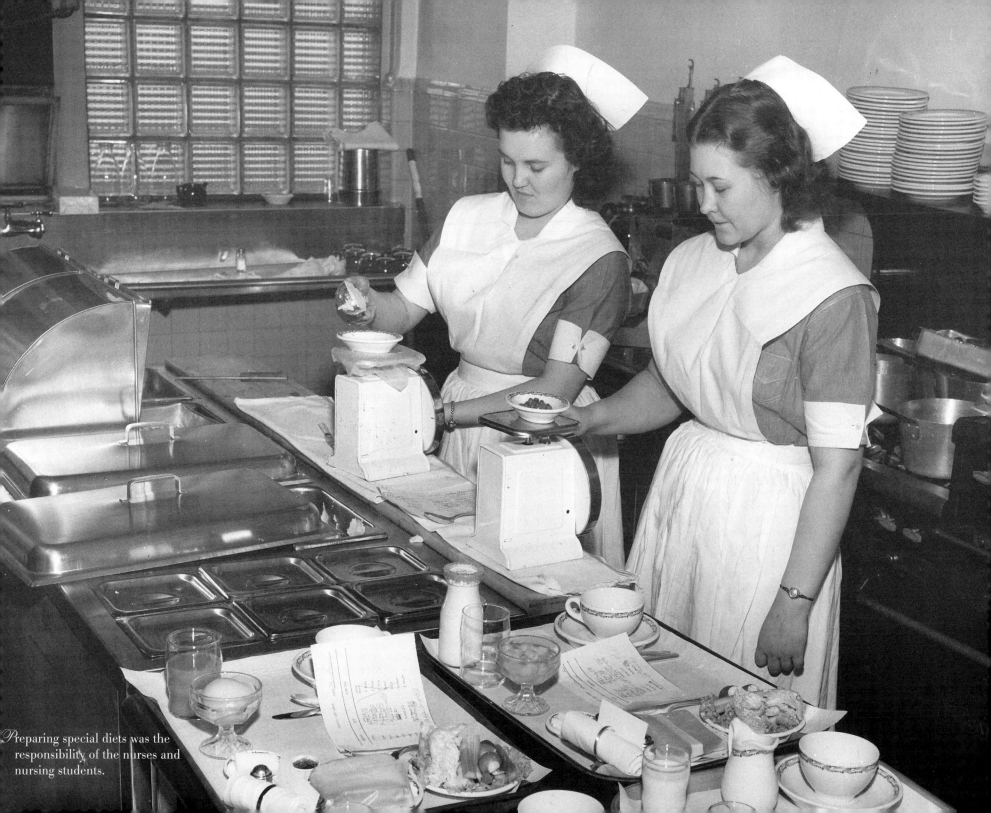

Preparing special diets was the responsibility of the nurses and nursing students.

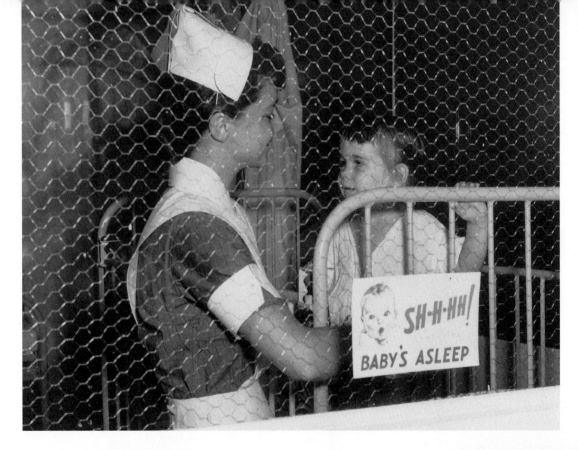

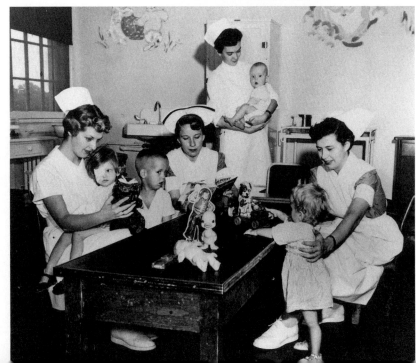

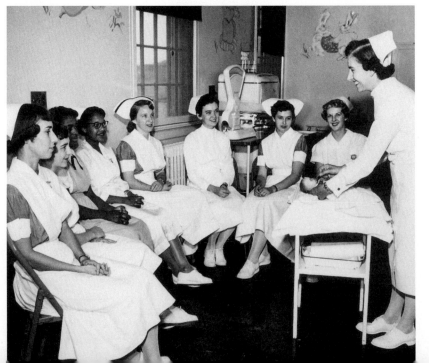

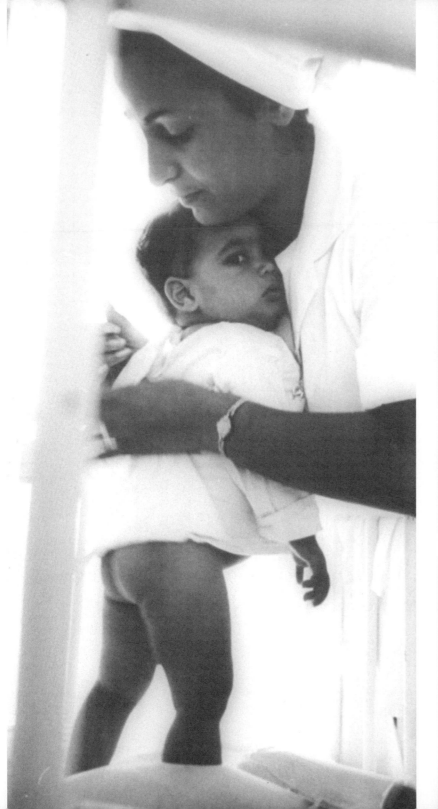
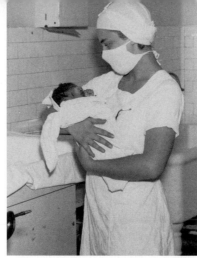
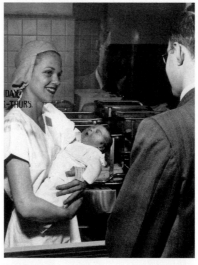
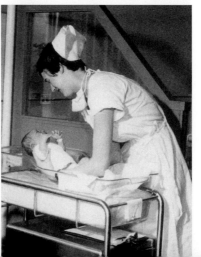
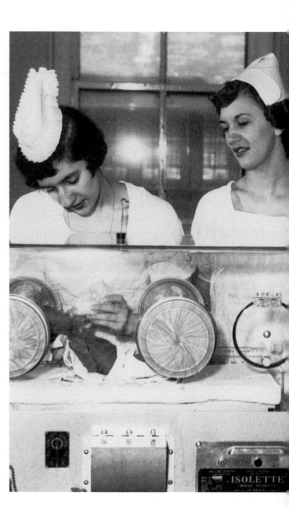

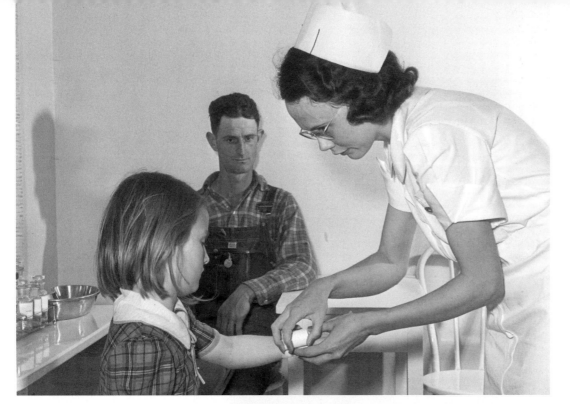

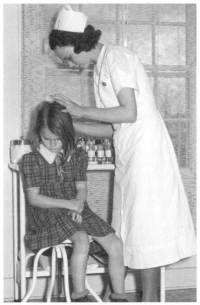

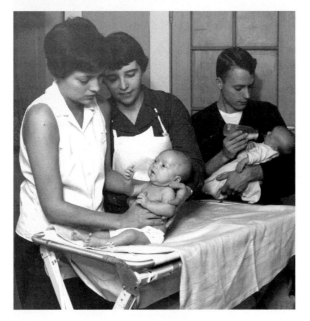

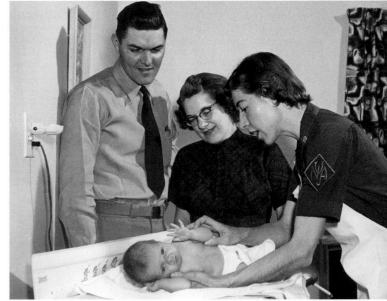

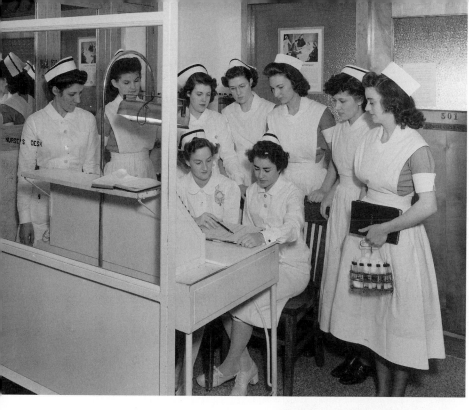

One night while I was on night duty as a junior student on a medical floor, an older patient had an insulin reaction. He got out of bed, and the night supervisor and I talked him into returning to bed. He was unable to void, so we had to catheterize him (since there were no orderlies on nights). His reaction to all of this was "the county fair was never like this." He recovered and didn't remember what had happened.

Marian Louise Goff
LOUISVILLE, KENTUCKY

Morning report.

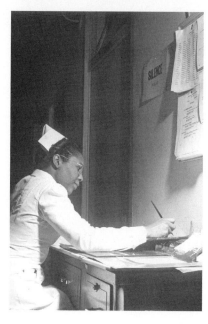

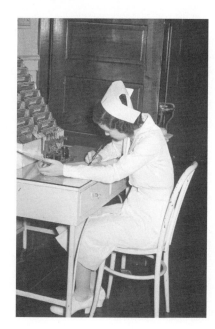

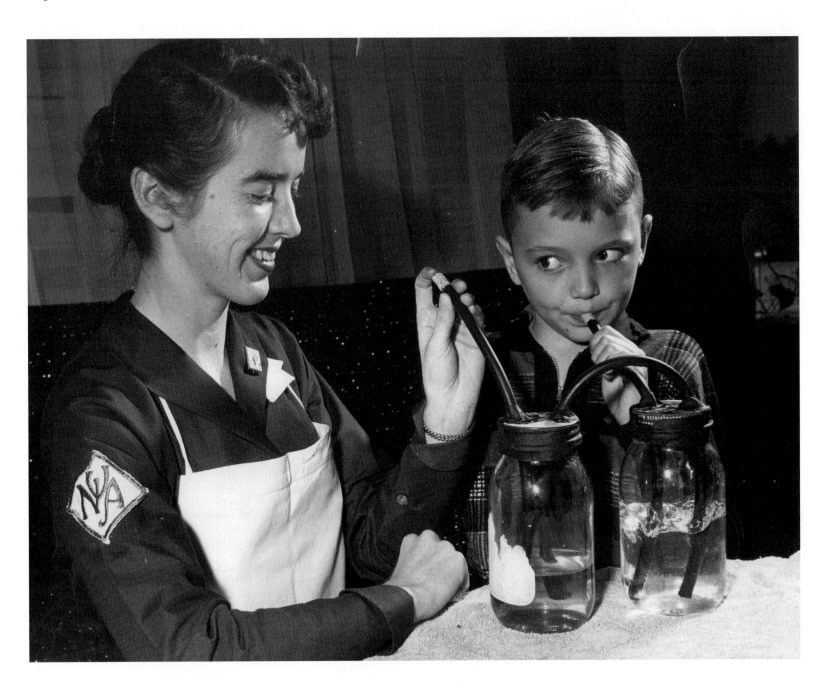

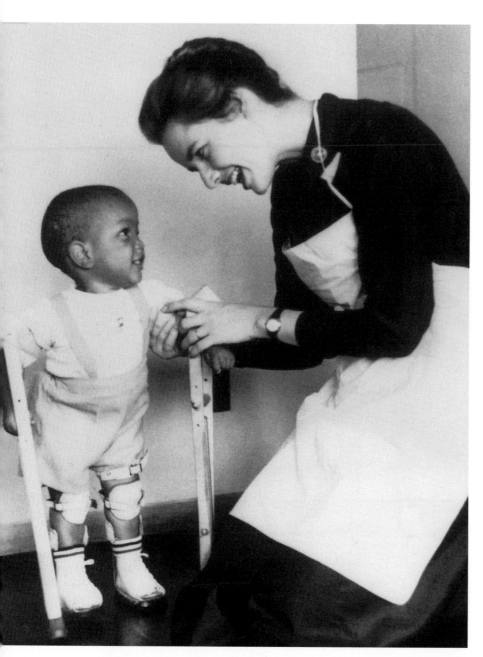

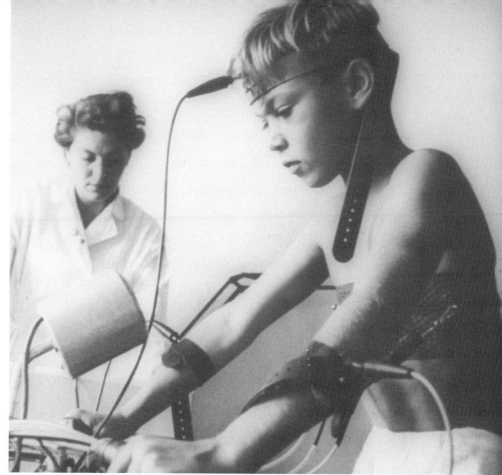

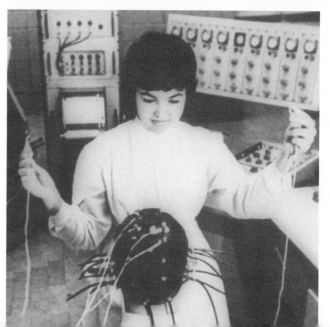

A nurse conducting an EEG on a patient.

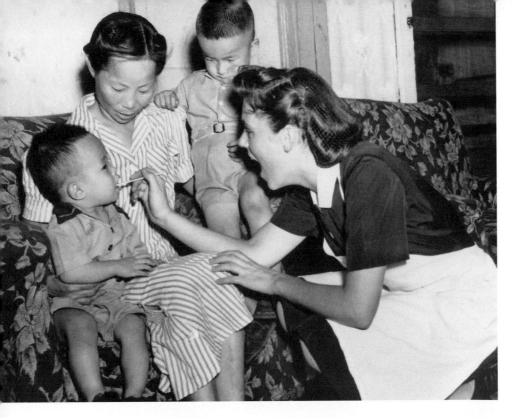

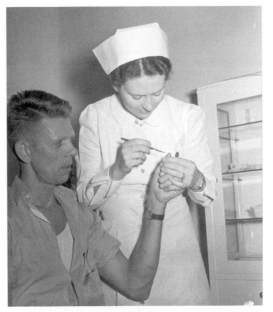

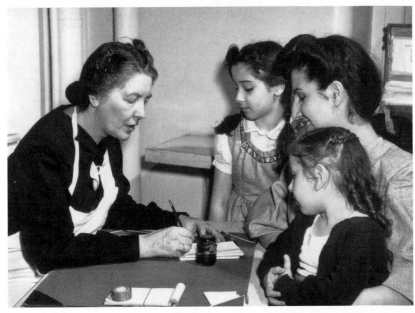

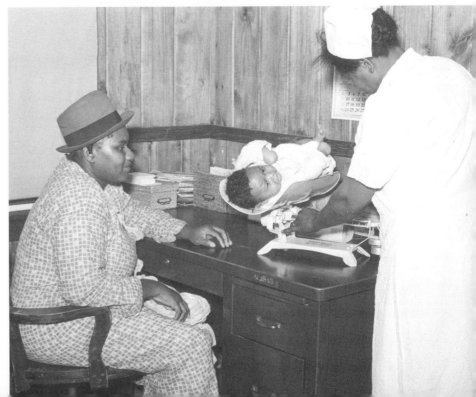

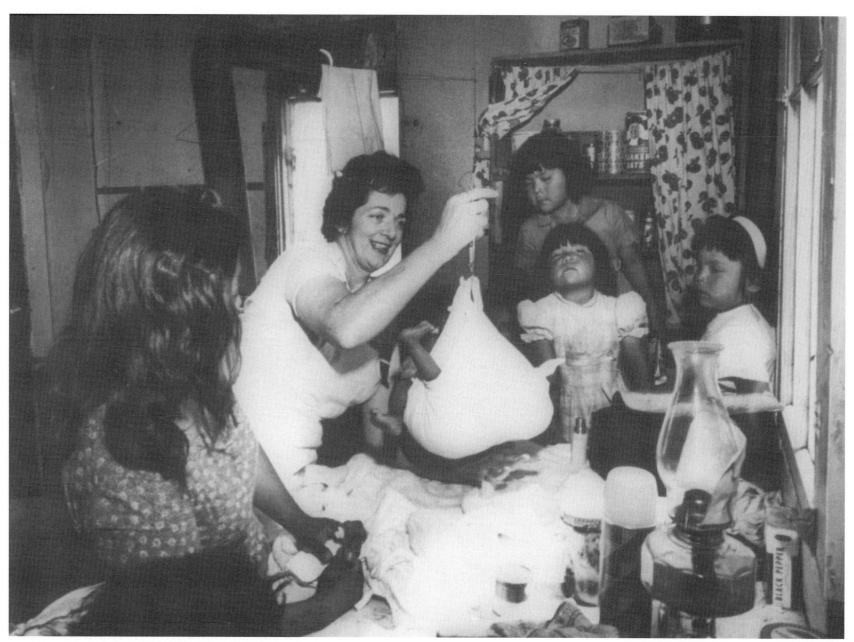

What does she weigh?

It was a hot, dry day in 1954 when I arrived on the train in the 112-degree heat to the small rural town in western Kansas. My new assignment was to replace the Sister on the third floor orthopedic unit, which included the overflow of medical, surgical, and pediatric medical patients. At the time I was in my early thirties, and I was out to convert the world. I had my big challenge.

On one very memorable evening I was just leaving the unit when the emergency room aide arrived on our unit with a young man covered with a sheet. I remember admitting Charles to a private room and starting to assess his condition when the aide said, "It's a burn victim."

The patient had been working in the oil fields and had been finished with his work for the day. His overalls were stained with large areas of oil, so the 19-year-old man had taken gasoline and had completed the stain removal. Then he lit a cigarette. His clothes ignited at that point. He received third-degree burns over most of his body—on his neck, arms, torso, legs, and back. Only his head and feet had been spared.

Our nurses and nurse's aides were instructed to care for him. His care included giving him a fruit drink to force fluids whenever someone passed his room. The roller bandages used to cover his burn areas were impregnated with a soothing ointment "to be left on until they fell off," according to the doctor's orders. He was placed

him on a Foster Frame to give him more comfort and change his position. He never lost consciousness. How we worried during the ensuing weeks about the healing under the bandages. One area on his left ankle was the only skin graft that he had.

Charles was a model patient during all these weeks. He knew we were there to help him heal and to return home. When all the bandages fell off, the healing process was progressing very well. We finally witnessed his dismissal. A year later he returned to visit us. Only a small scar on his left ankle was evident from this horrible gasoline burn. How we all rejoiced with Charles on his recovery.

Sister Jeanette Thelen
Fond-du-Lac, Wisconsin

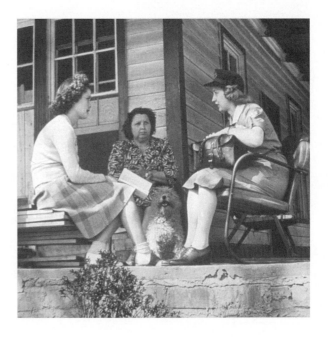

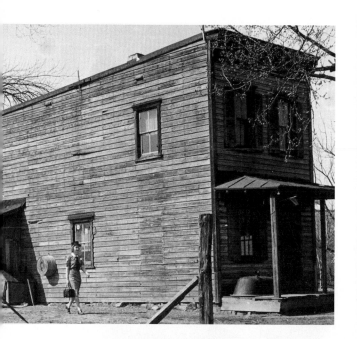

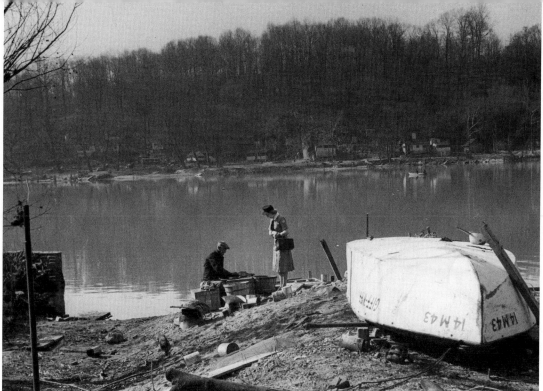

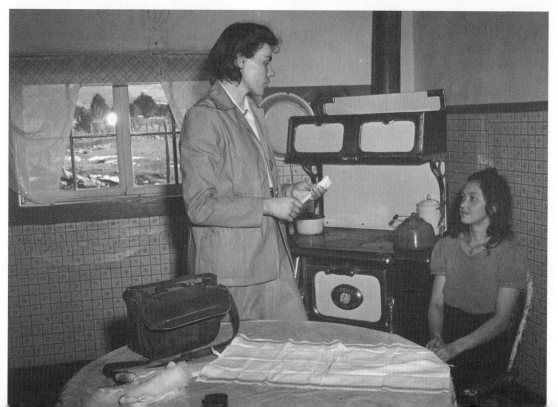

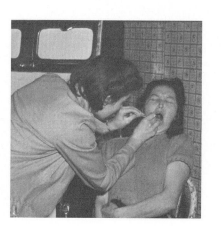

84

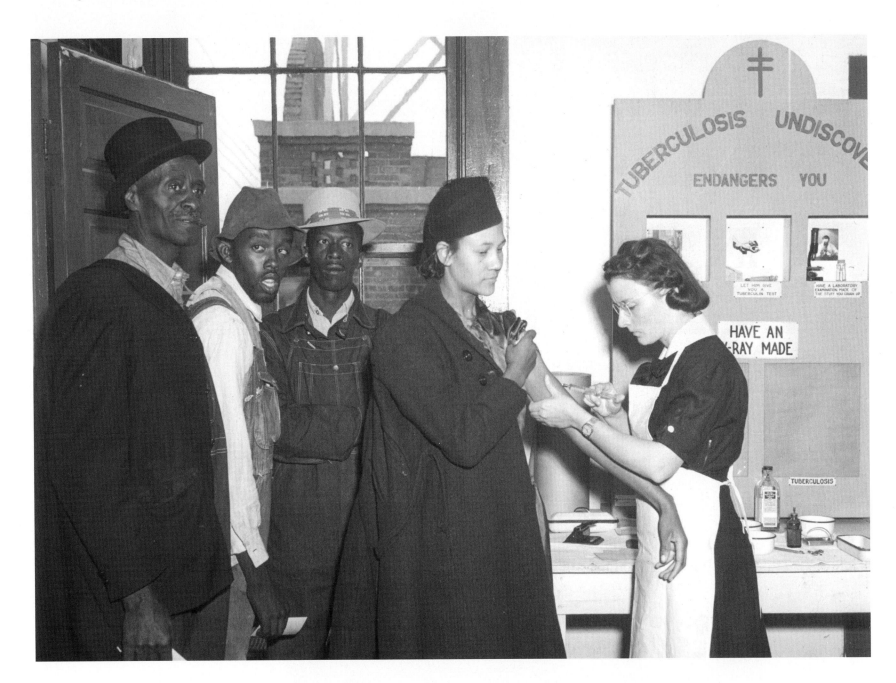

Mrs. Richard Nixon helps the Visiting Nurse Association (now MedStar
Health Visiting Nurse Association serving Washington D.C., Maryland,
and Northern Virginia) of Washington D.C. celebrate its 55th anniversary.

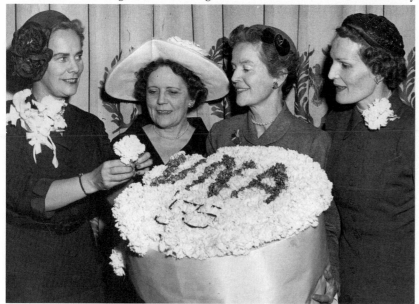

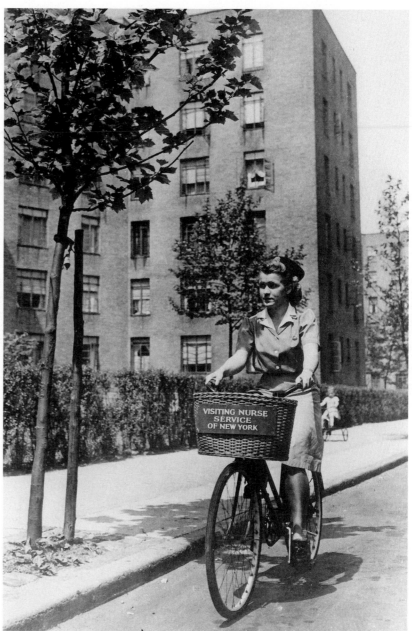

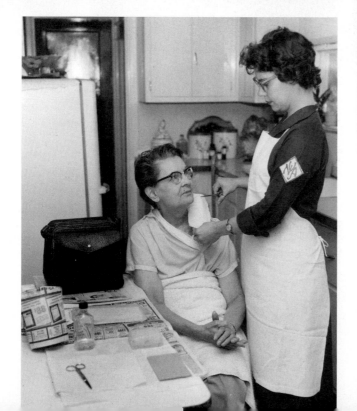

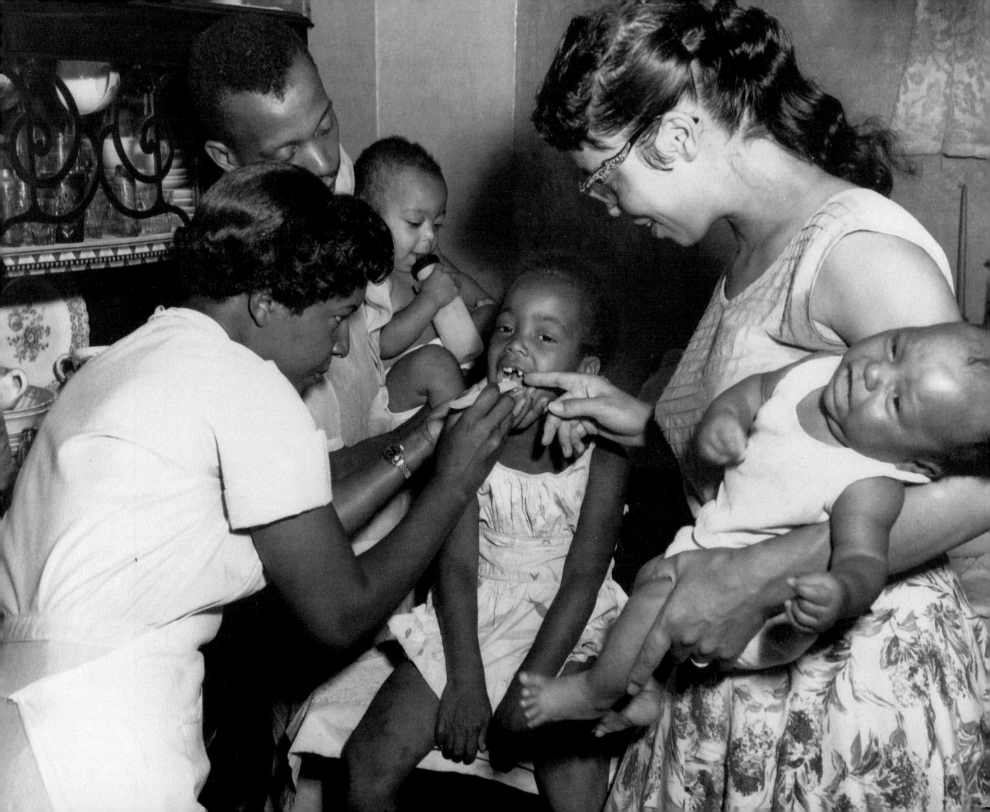

1960s

1960

The first birth control pill is made available to the public.

Medical specialization flourishes throughout the decade with the establishment of units for coronary care, surgical and medical intensive care, burns, dialysis, oncology, and the like, stimulating specialization in nursing.

The world population reaches 3 billion.

Chubby Checkers' "The Twist" starts a dance craze.

1961

The incidence of polio in the United States drops by 95%.

The Berlin Wall is built to stop the escape of refugees from East Berlin to West Berlin.

The invasion of Cuba at the Bay of Pigs fails.

President Kennedy forms the Peace Corps.

Soviet cosmonaut Yuri Gagarin conducts the first manned space flight.

1962

American military nurses become involved in the Vietnam efforts.

The United States and Soviet Union come close to war because of Soviet nuclear missiles in Cuba.

John Glenn becomes the first American to orbit the Earth.

1963

President Kennedy is assassinated in Dallas.

Martin Luther King, Jr., delivers his "I Have a Dream" speech.

Michael DeBakey uses the first artificial heart to sustain blood circulation during surgery.

The Beatles sing "I Want To Hold Your Hand."

New Hampshire runs the first state lottery in the United States.

1964

North Vietnam attacks U.S. destroyers in the Gulf of Tonkin.

President Johnson begins his "war on poverty" with the Economic Opportunity Act, which provides funds for vocational training, encourages community action programs, and establishes a domestic peace corps.

Although the Surgeon General releases a report linking smoking to lung cancer, the popularity of cigarette smoking in the United States increases.

The Civil Rights Bill is passed and calls for an end to discrimination.

President Johnson signs the Medicare Act into law.

1965

President Johnson orders the bombing of North Vietnam.

Marine troops land in Vietnam in March, and by June a full-scale offensive begins.

Dr. Henry Silver, a pediatrician, and Dr. Loretta Ford, a public health nurse, collaborate to establish the first pediatric nurse practitioner program.

At the University of Michigan, a "teach-in" is held to protest the Vietnam War, heralding the beginning of the student antiwar movement.

Malcolm X, a leader of civil rights and black power, is shot and killed in New York City.

1966

By February, 300 Army, Navy, and Air Force nurses are serving in Vietnam.

Masters and Johnson publish the report *Human Sexual Response*.

Congress authorizes commissions in the regular Army for male nurses.

The Beatles record "Yesterday."

1967

Christiaan Barnard performs the first human heart transplant.

Antiwar sentiment increases in the United States.

A fire on the U.S. Apollo rocket during launch tests kills three astronauts.

Colorado becomes the first state to legalize abortion.

Massachusetts General Hospital establishes a nurse-staffed Medical Station at Logan International Hospital. The station has two-way audiovisual communication with the hospital.

The rock musical *Hair* opens in New York.

1968

Martin Luther King, Jr., and Robert Kennedy are assassinated.

First Philadelphia Bank installs the first cash-dispensing machine.

1969

Neil Armstrong and Edwin Aldrin land on the moon and explore the plain known as the *Sea of Tranquility*.

The Woodstock music festival reigns for 4 days in the Catskill Mountains.

The first in vitro fertilization of an egg occurs.

In June, the United States begins troop reductions in Vietnam.

Sesame Street debuts on public television.

88

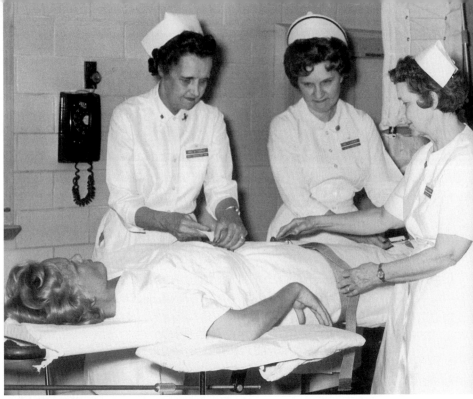

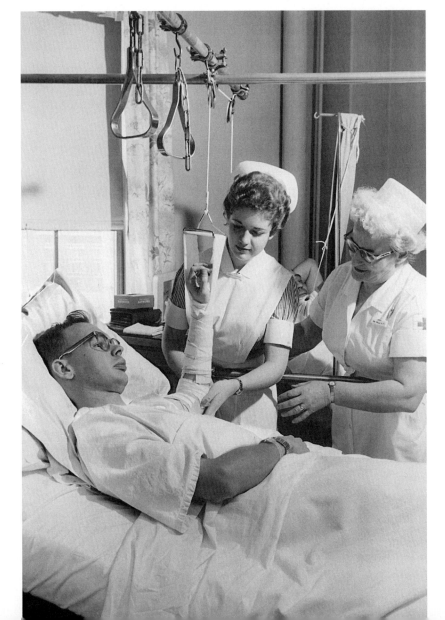

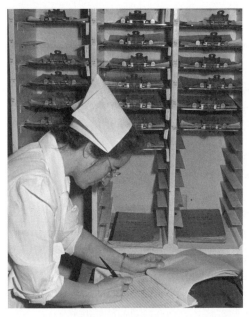

Teaching, mentoring, and
always charting.

I remember "specialing" Steven who had suffered a head injury following an auto accident. His treatment consisted of using a hypothermia machine to control his body temperature. The machine was large and had two chambers that needed alcohol added periodically. It pumped the alcohol through the coils in two rubber mats that were on top of and under the patient. A rectal thermometer was in place. As Steven's temperature went too low, we would turn the machine off, and when the temperature went too high, we would turn the machine back on again. This balancing act was continuous until his condition stabilized.

Linda Bowers
WINTER GARDEN, FLORIDA

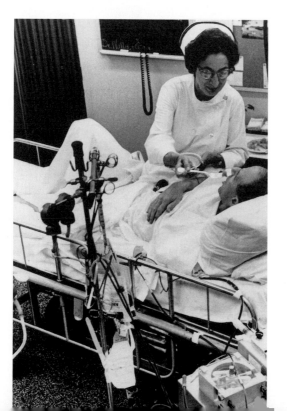

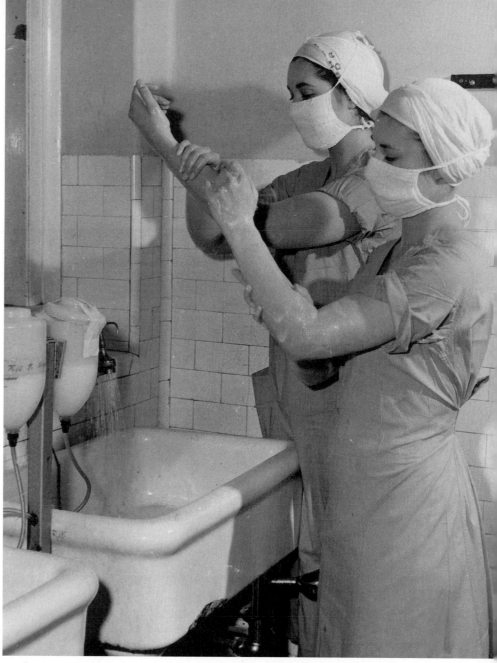

Always—a 10-minute scrub before entering the operating room.

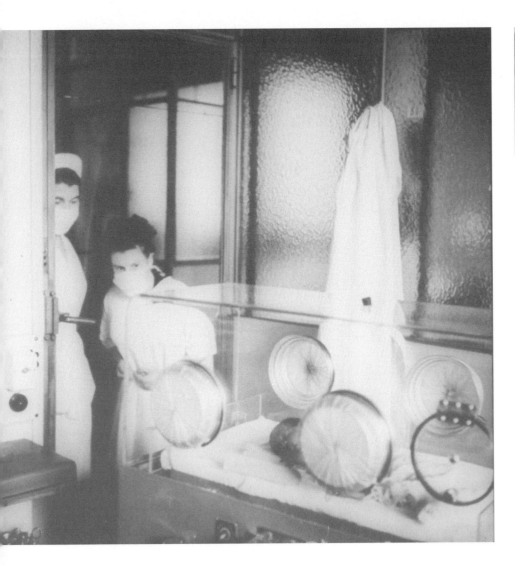

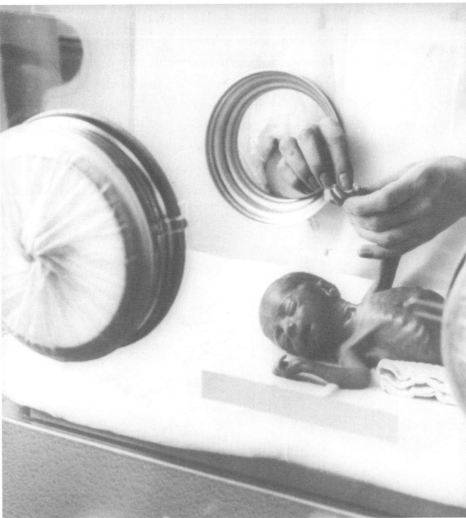

Tender caring for this small miracle.

I was a nursing student in 1961 in a diploma program run by a small-town hospital. This was before the time of intensive care units and even before the use of code blues within the hospital system. As our instructor handed out our assignments, we were all eager to get down to the business of nursing. My assignment was a 43-year-old male who had been in a knife fight 2 days earlier. He had numerous wounds that were suppurative and draining. His temperature was 106.5 and BP was 80/40. He was on antibiotics and an antipyretic and had an intravenous and continuous ice packs. In today's world this man would have been in the ICU.

When I entered the room, I saw a comatose male who was so tall that he stretched from the top to the bottom of the bed and was so wide that he almost stretched from side to side. I began my assessment with vital signs: temperature 107, pulse 140, blood pressure 80/40. Skin was cold and clammy, and he was perspiring. Abdomen was distended. His multiple wound dressings all needed changing. I notified my instructor. Beginning students did not care for IVs, so the instructor notified the RN about the vital signs.

I identified my first goal: to bring the temperature down. I knew that this man was close to death, but I was bound and determined that I was going to save him. After all, I was a nurse, and this was why I had become a nurse.

I worked with this man for 2 hours, sponging, bathing, using ice packs, changing dressings, changing the bed and positioning him. Finally, I was done. I felt satisfied but worried. I felt that I had done all that I could do. I left the room and went to help other students.

About 10 minutes later, I heard the RN in the hall saying that he had died. I was devastated. My fellow students all gathered around me as I burst into tears. I couldn't believe that he died after all I had done for him. Later, I was to realize that nursing was not only helping one to live but also helping one to die with dignity.

Marti Whiting
ALBUQUERQUE, NEW MEXICO

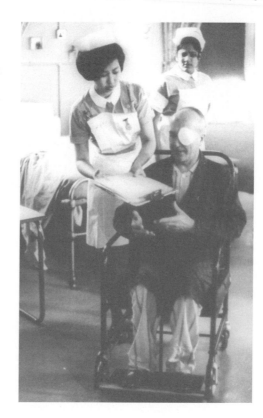

91

92

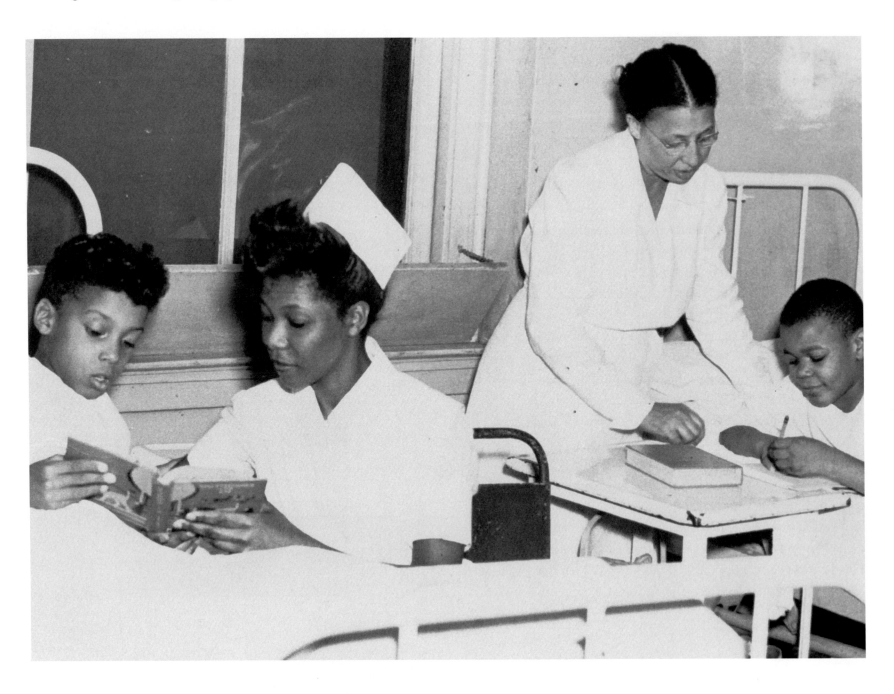

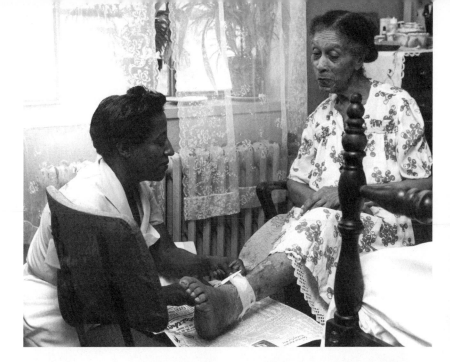

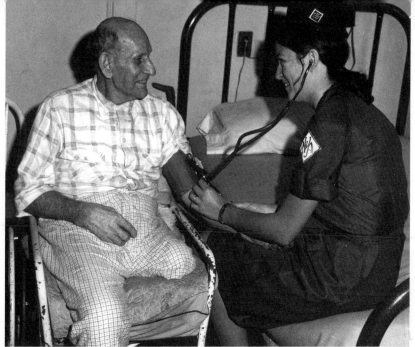

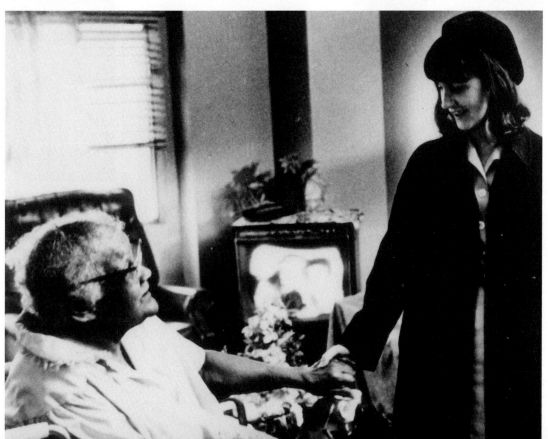

The healing touch.

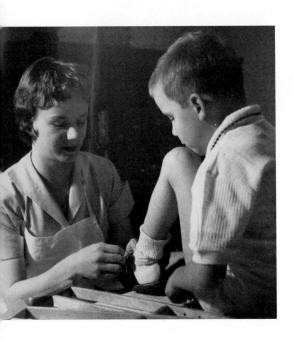

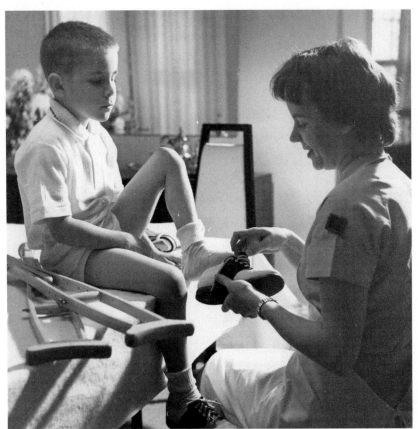

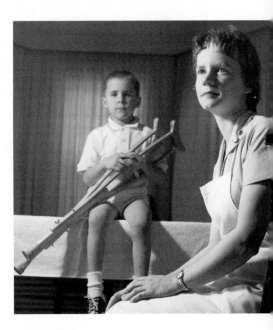

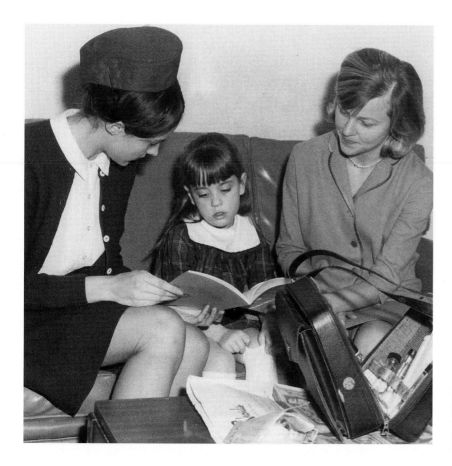

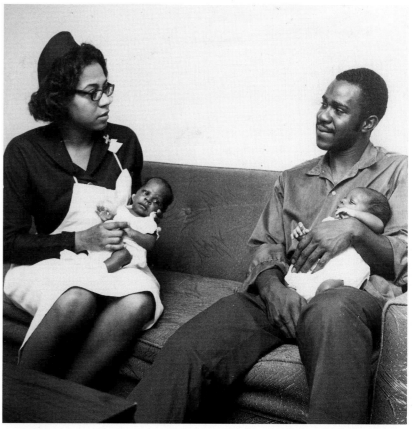

Listen, teach, and listen again.

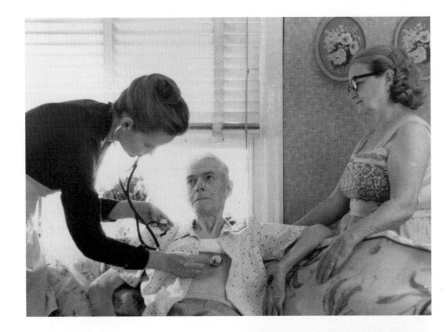

96

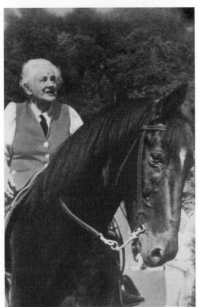

Mary Breckinridge, founder of the
Frontier Nursing Service, on
her horse Babette.

My Great Aunt Juel had a passion for stories about the Old South, and her all-time favorite was *Gone with the Wind*, which she took me to see on more than one occasion. I remember very clearly doing the dishes with her one night, and she turned to me with tears in her eyes and said, "I so wanted you to be a Melanie, but I fear you will be a Scarlet O'Hara." At that time I didn't understand.

Aunt Juel and Uncle Joe had no children, so as a child growing up I spent many days with them. It was just after my sixteenth birthday that my Aunt Juel first began encouraging me to become a nurse. Because they offered to pay for my schooling and because my babysitter income was meager, the decision became easy. My grandmother was an old-time nurse, and my knowledge of nurses and nursing was limited to her use of old-time remedies.

Neither my Aunt Juel nor my grandmother lived to see me graduate from nursing school. In the early part of my career, I did not appreciate the wisdom of either of these two influential women. But now, some 38 years later, I truly believe that during my rich nursing career, I have come to embrace many of the qualities of "a Melanie." As I look back I thank my Aunt Juel for her deep love and for giving me the precious gift of nursing.

Linda Ann Melley
LAKESIDE, PENNSYLVANIA

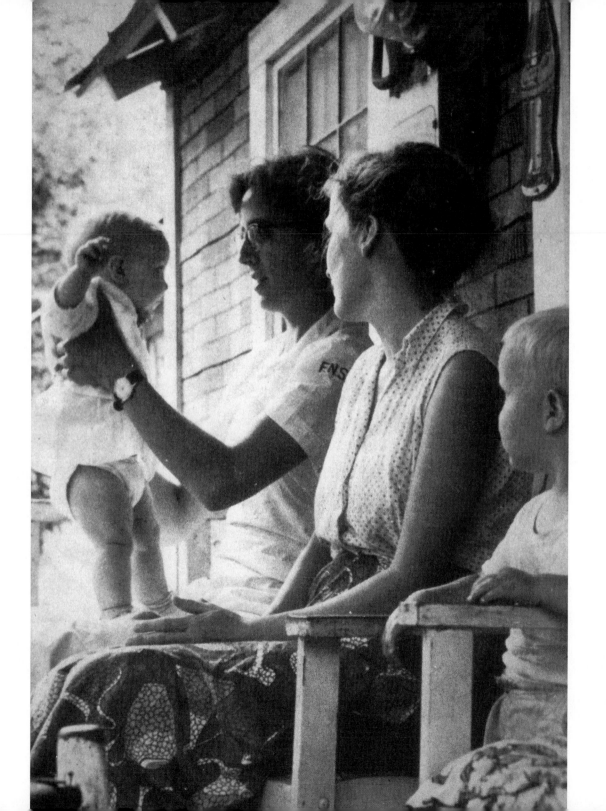

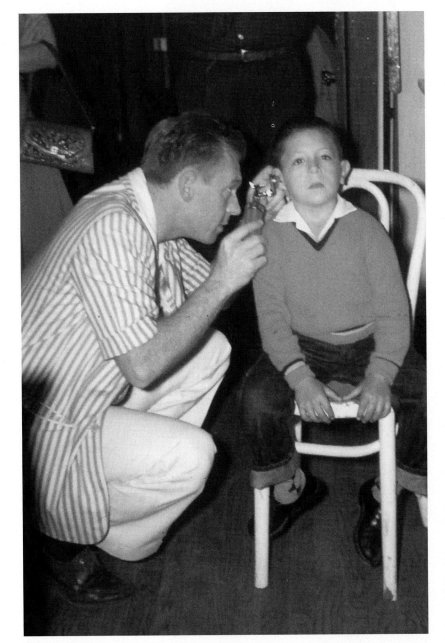

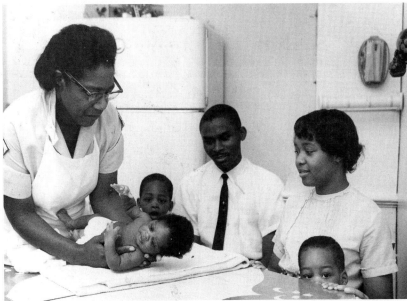

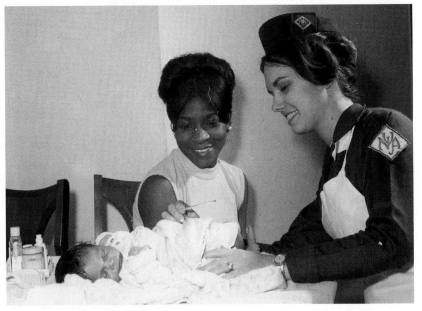

Care at a Frontier Nursing Service clinic.

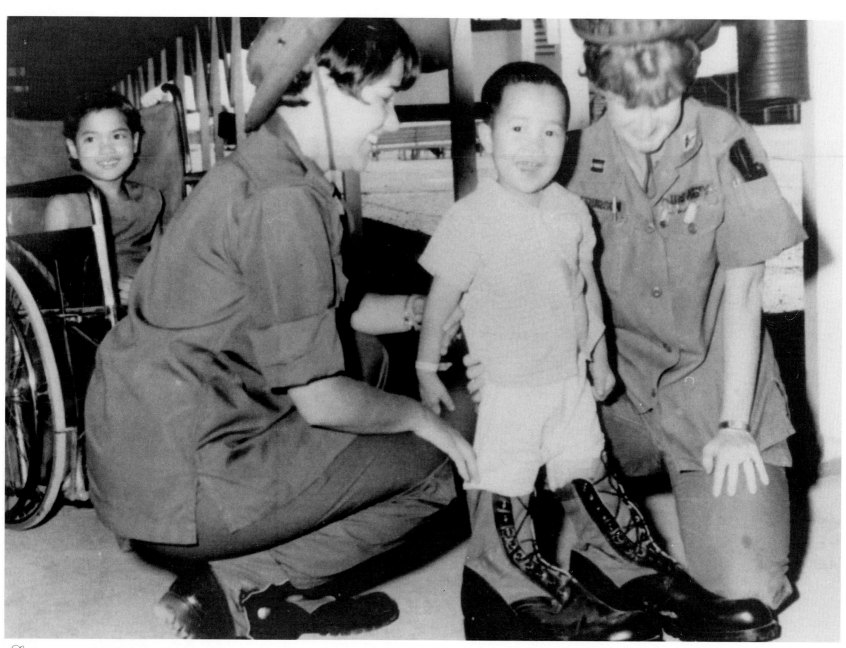

Some very big shoes to fill.

*D*uring the Vietnam War more than 7,500 nurses served. Mass casualities. Amazing how much I aged in just 6 months.

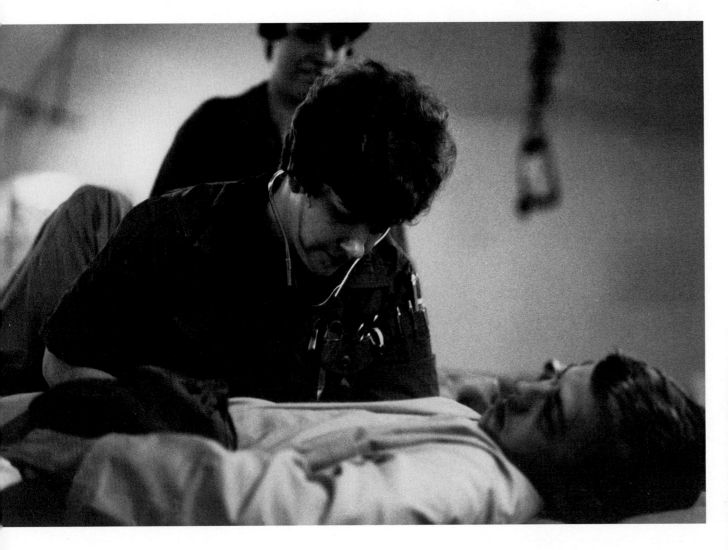

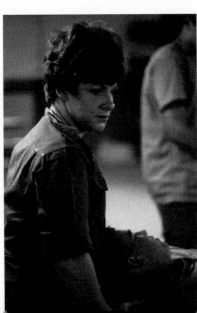

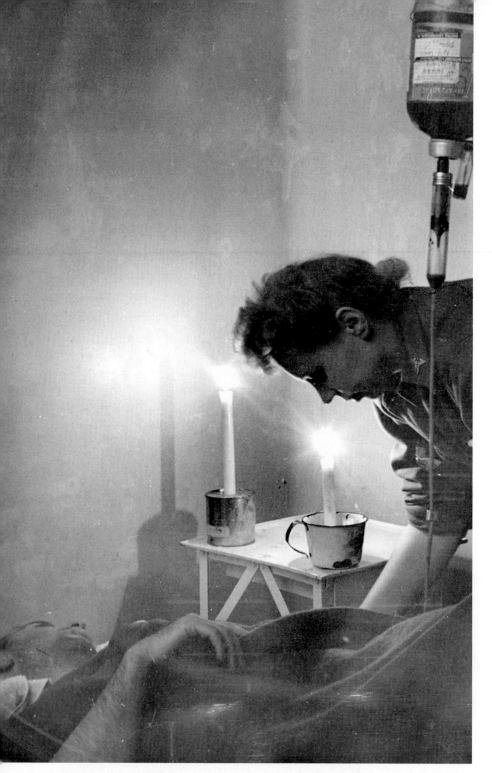

*N*urses went to Vietnam for hundreds of personal reasons. Patients needed care, and nurses volunteered to provide it. We were not drafted. We asked to be there.

We arrived with some civilian experience and many delusions of grandeur. The military tried to prepare us with facts for what we would see, but it was impossible to tell us how we were going to feel and how much impact it would have on our lives.

As a new arrival, barely checked in and processed, I was off and running with 36 patients from the first Chinook (chopper). Before we could finish caring for those patients, another chopper arrived with 36 more. And they just kept coming. We realized it was all up to us. No one was coming around "later" to tell us what to do.

The nurses in Vietnam quickly learned to assess, do, and move on. There was no looking back. The decisions made and actions taken were nothing like the civilian nursing world we came from. We triaged and proceeded to intubate, insert chest tubes, amputate limbs, and do whatever else was required for our patients to survive. There were no bad nurses in Vietnam.

With the constant arrival of new patients, we could never catch up, but there were some things to feel good about. A lot of patients lived because of what we did. Our role was much bigger than our training prepared us for, but, being nurses, the nurses in Vietnam, did it, and did it well.

Any Nurse from the Army Nurse Corps

101

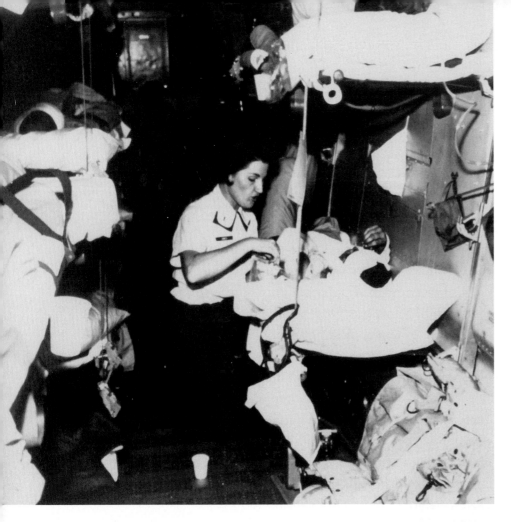

I finally got to Chu Lai to begin my year in country. One of the few patients I remember was a young GI who got hit by a land mine and had a traumatic above-the-knee amputation of his right leg. My head nurse told me he had the "million dollar" wound and was going to be shipped out the next day. I was assigned to change his bed and reinforce his dressings. When I went to turn him over, his dressing and bed was covered with maggots. I quickly turned him back and ran to the head nurse, shocked by what I had found. I was told, "Oh, that is okay. They will eat the dead flesh, and the docs will clean him up when he gets to Japan. Welcome to combat nursing, Anna Marie!"

Anna Marie Rutallie
INDIANAPOLIS, INDIANA

When a young man's life was on the line, the evacuation flight to Japan seemed to take so long.

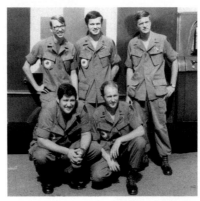

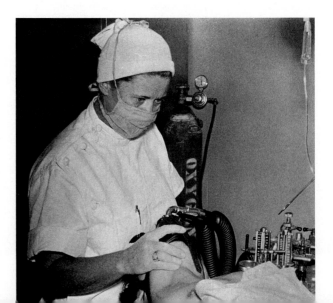

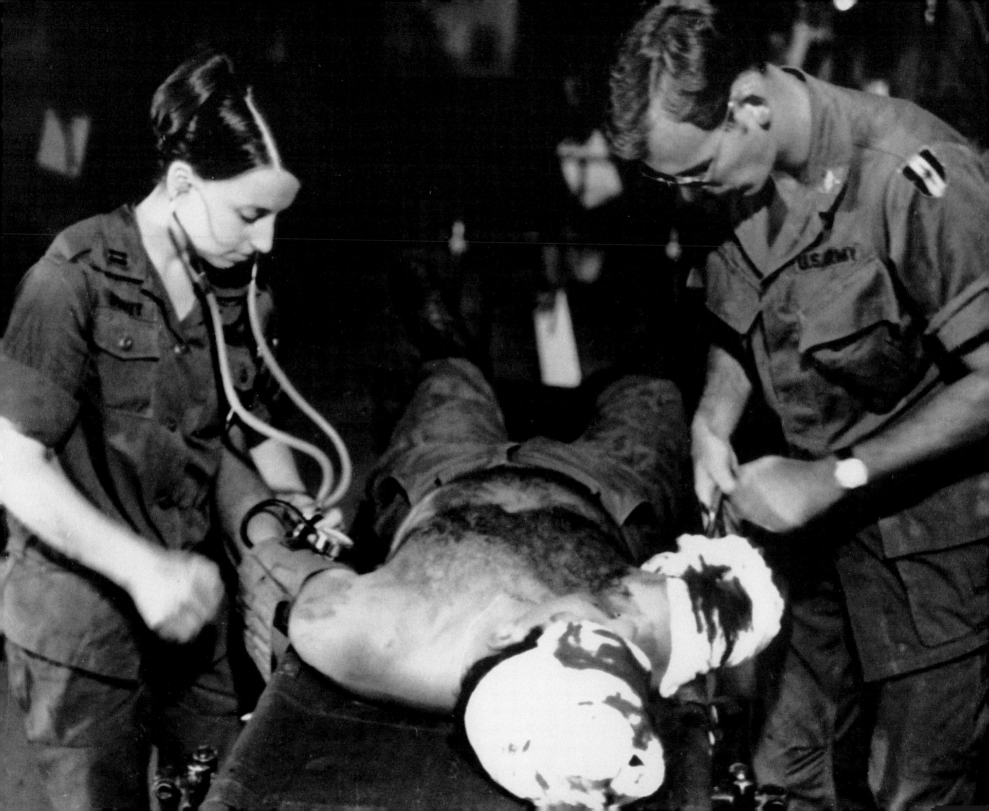

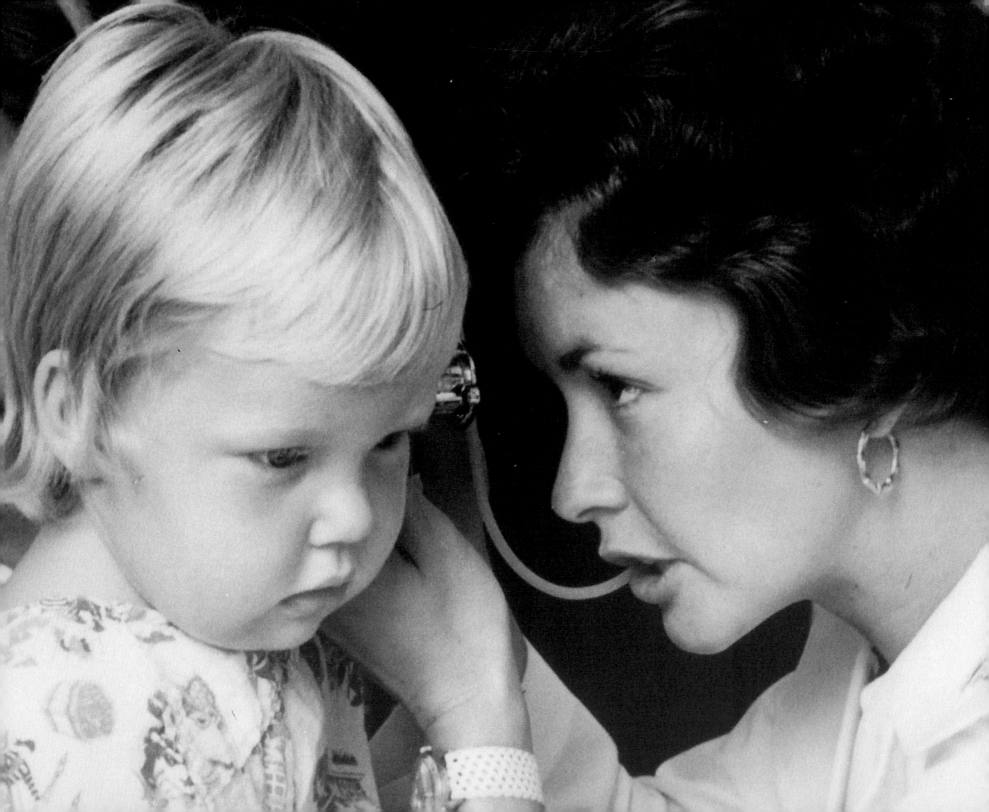

_1970s_

1970

The computerized axial tomography (CAT) machine is first used.

A total of 126 runners show up for the first New York Marathon.

National Guardsmen open fire, killing four and injuring eight students at Kent State University in Ohio during a Vietnam War protest.

CIA activity in Laos is exposed.

The Environmental Protection Agency (EPA) is created by Congress to control air and water pollution; the first Earth Day is observed.

The Beatles break up.

1971

Intel develops the first microprocessor chip.

IBM introduces the first "memory disk," today called the _floppy disk_.

The Twenty-Sixth Amendment lowers the voting age from 21 to 18 in the United States.

A total of 26 rural health clinic sites in Alaska are video-linked by NASA's Applied Technology Satellites to larger, physician-staffed facilities.

The United States begins to spend millions of dollars on the development and distribution of a vaccine to prevent the swine flu, which never materializes.

Cigarette sales top $540 billion despite a partial ban on cigarette advertising.

1972

The pesticide DDT is banned in the United States.

President Nixon makes historic visits to China and the Soviet Union.

Arab guerrillas murder 11 Israeli athletes at the Munich Olympics.

Five men with surveillance equipment and cameras are arrested inside the new Democratic National Headquarters, marking the beginning of the Watergate scandal and the end of Nixon's presidency.

The Senate approves the Equal Rights Amendment, but it fails to be ratified by the required number of states.

1973

OPEC raises oil prices by 70% and again by 130%, precipitating the oil crisis.

Direct American involvement in Vietnam ends. Bombings of Cambodia continue in an effort to retrieve prisoners of war.

In _Roe v. Wade_, the Supreme Court rules that women have the unrestricted right to abortion in the first trimester of pregnancy.

The First National Conference on the Classification of Nursing Diagnoses is held in St. Louis.

1974

In an effort to conserve auto fuel, President Nixon signs an act limiting highway speeds to 55 mph.

President Nixon, faced with possible impeachment as a result of the Watergate scandal, becomes the first U.S. president to resign from office.

Inflation is climbing around the world; in the United States, prices rise more than 10%, and unemployment tops 9%.

Henry Heimlich describes the Heimlich maneuver.

1975

Clinicians at the University of California successfully treat the first neonatal patient using extracorporeal life support (ECMO).

The last American troops leave Vietnam.

Bill Gates and Paul Allen start Microsoft.

1976

The U.S. spacecraft Vikings 1 and 2 successfully touch down on Mars' surface and transmit data back to Earth.

The first Apple Computer is built.

North and South Vietnam unite as one country.

1977

Balloon angioplasty surgery is pioneered.

Elvis Presley is found dead at age 42 at Graceland in Memphis.

1978

Louise Brown, the first test tube baby, is born in England.

The U.S. government recognizes the People's Republic of China.

Some 98% of all U.S. households have a television.

Jim Jones and over 900 followers drink Kool-Aid spiked with cyanide in a mass suicide in Jonestown, Guyana.

1979

The smallpox eradication program of the World Health Organization is completed.

Three Mile Island nuclear plant near Harrisburg, Pennsylvania, suffers a partial meltdown.

Cellular phones are introduced in Japan.

The U.S. space probes Voyager 1 and 2 reach Jupiter.

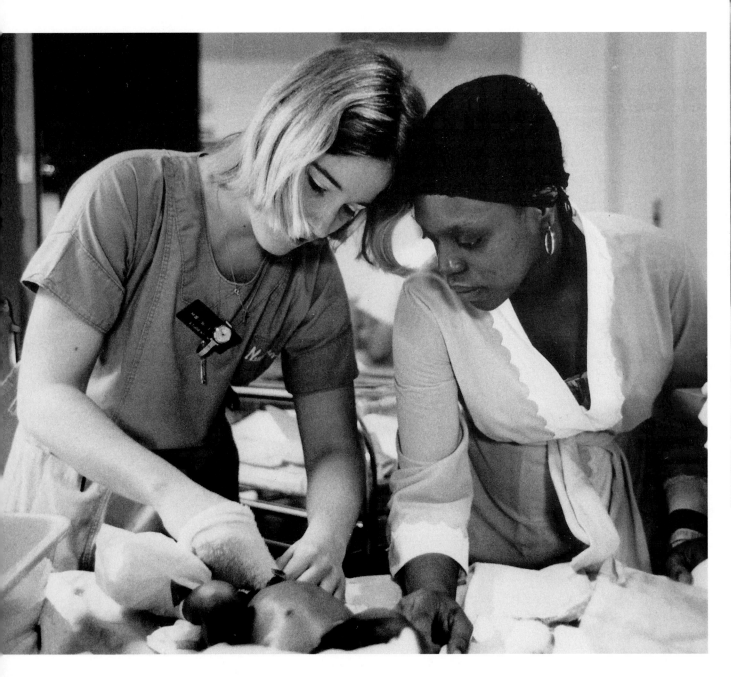

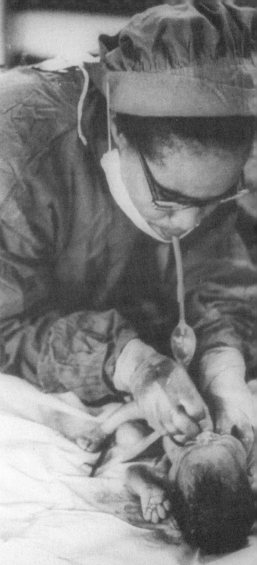

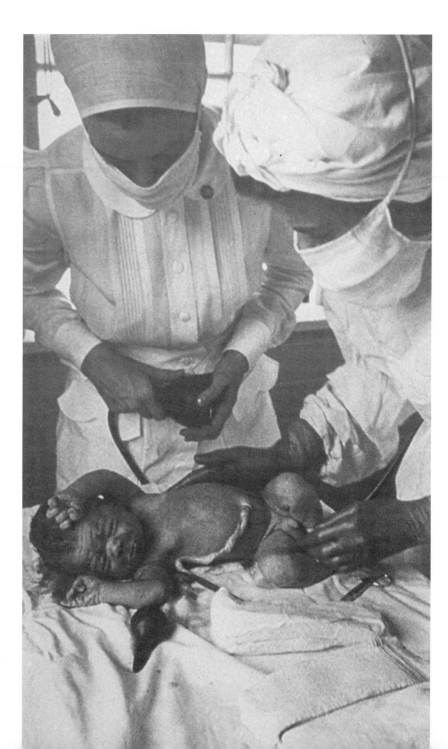

*I*n 1974, I became the first perinatal outreach educator funded by a grant from the National Foundation March of Dimes. I traveled in seven states, including Colorado, Wyoming, Montana, western Nebraska, Kansas, South Dakota, and New Mexico, to teach nurses and doctors in our referral area to recognize and stabilize sick newborns.

As two physicians and I began teaching a 2-day workshop, an "older" doctor (about 60 years old) put his arm around me and said, "Honey, you're too young. You couldn't possibly know what you're doing." Since I was an "ambassador" for the hospital and the grant, I suppressed my initial response and tactfully responded, "I hope at the end of the next 2 days, you won't be able to say that." At the completion of the workshop, the physician said, "You know, honey, you do know what you're doing!"

Because of the outreach education of nurses and physicians, babies were warm, oxygenated, normoglycemic, and stable when the transport team arrived. Earlier referral of at-risk mothers and babies coupled with their more stabilized condition has been linked to the decrease in neonatal mortality rate in Colorado: dropping from 13.4 to 6.9 between 1971 and 1978.

Sandra L. Gardner
Aurora, Colorado

107

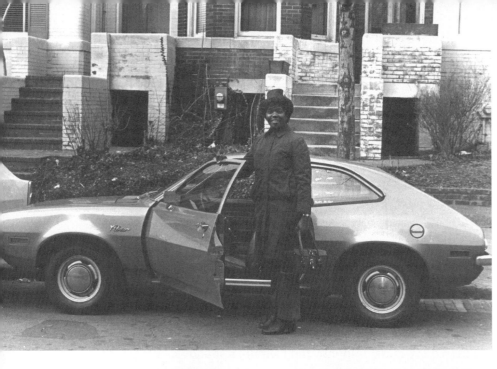

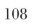

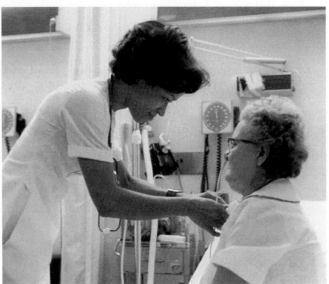

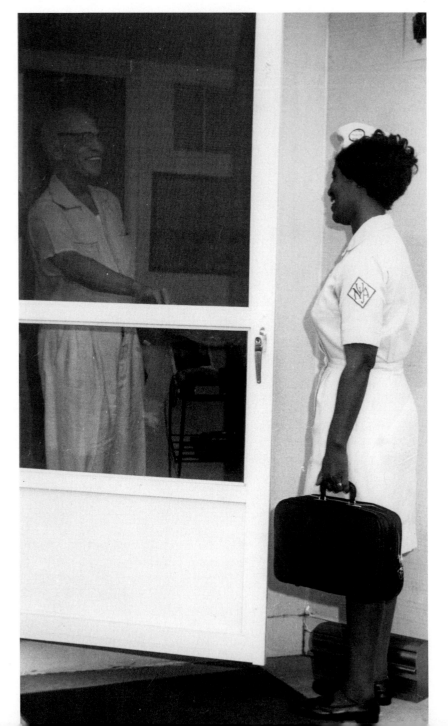

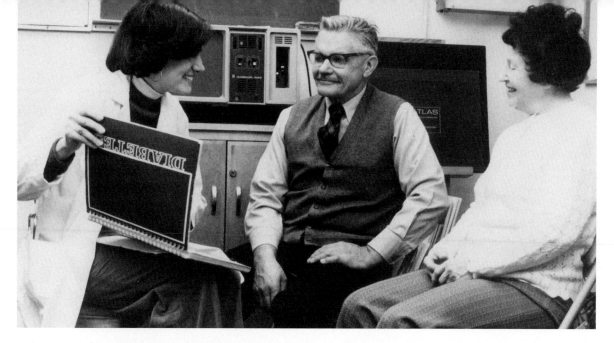

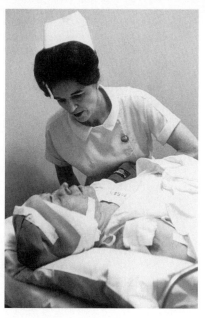

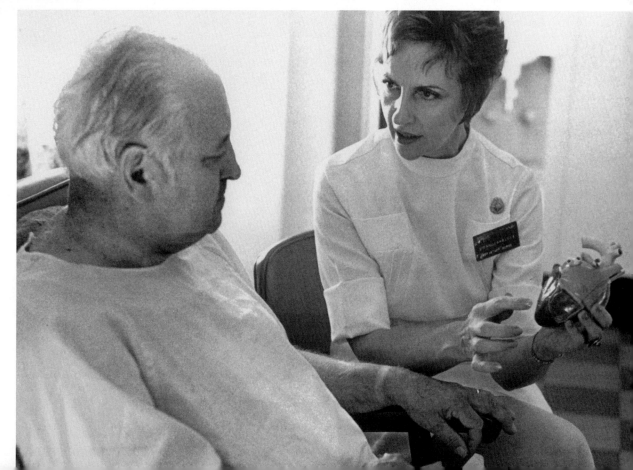

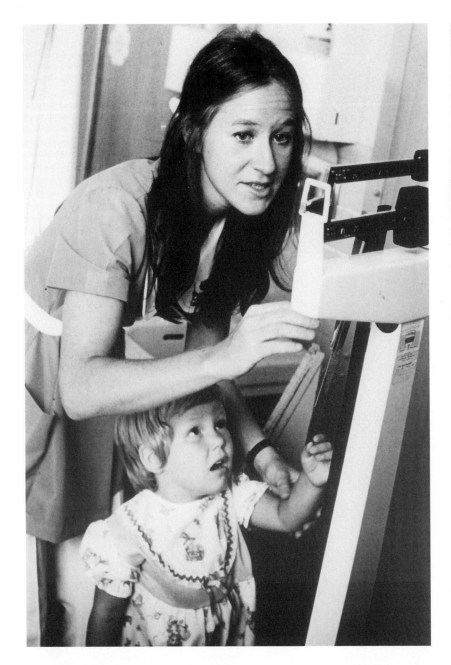

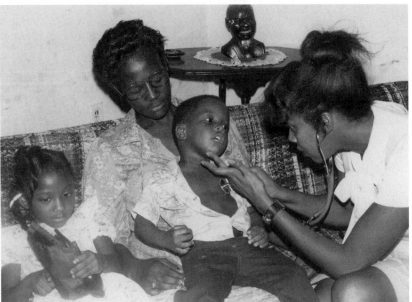

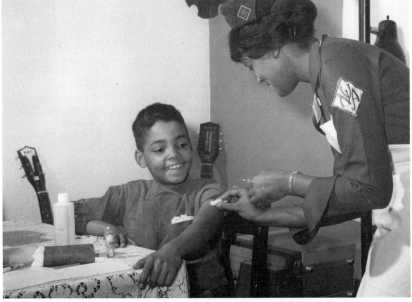

It was long ago, in the early 1970s, but I recall the event as if it were yesterday. The summer night was hot, and somehow this seemed appropriate for my first shift as a pediatric nurse. I was responsible for the medications and treatments for 27 ill and injured children with surgical needs. As a recent nursing diploma recipient, I felt equal to the task. I felt confident, poised, and energetic, until I saw him—the child in Room 3006. He was six, frail, bedridden, and dying. In the 1970s, pediatric care was different, seemingly antiquated, and outcomes were more dismal for children who had large abdominal tumors. His was large and visible.

The time I could spend with the sick charges on my watch was limited. I ran from room to room to keep medication administration on time. It was not uncommon then for sicker children to be placed in "windowed" rooms so that nurses, as they scurried from one task to another, could provide ongoing monitoring and assessment via glances using peripheral vision when near the rooms. This small child was alone in his windowed room and was described by staff as the "difficult one." I soon experienced why he had been labeled "difficult"—he frequently pushed his call button. The annoying buzz became a reminder to busy nurses, including myself, that he needed something—the buzzing was constant. When asked, the child in Room 3006 would deny that he pushed the button; however, I observed tears in his large brown eyes. I had never seen a dying child, and I wasn't quite sure what aspect of "holistic" nursing I needed to provide for my sickest charge. His medication and treatments were few; he hadn't eaten over many shifts. His I&O was dismal.

At the end of my first shift I passed his room, feeling that I had somehow failed in my delivery of care. He was irritable, whining, and

sad. I sat with him and held his small hand, which still cradled the call button. Our topic of conversation was unusual—fruit he said was good. We settled on what he thought was the best—a purple plum. He thought he could eat one, his voice softened, he closed his tired eyelids, and fell asleep. I stayed a while, tucked him in, left the call button in his hand, and went home. The next day, my second shift as a pediatric nurse, I bounced onto the ward, and made a beeline for Room 3006. I placed the largest, most purple plum on the nightstand, sat on the vacant, stripped bed in Room 3006, and wept.

Kathy Haley
Worthington, Ohio

111

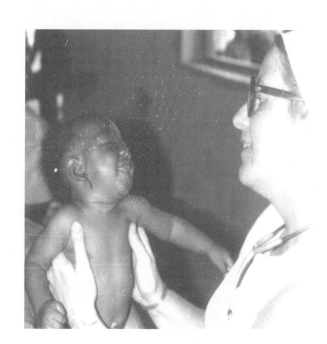

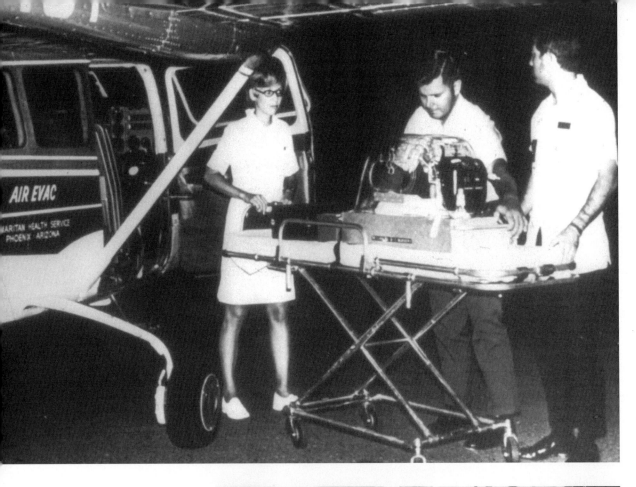

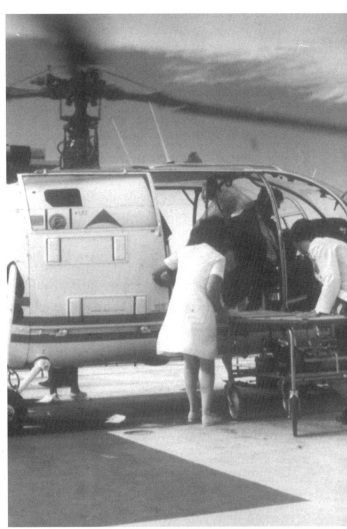

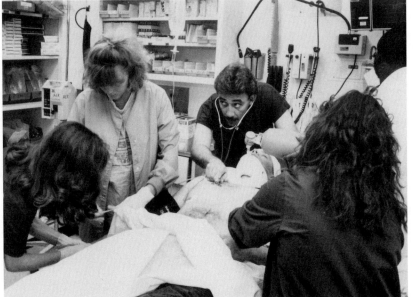

In the community, the home, the hospital, schools, and in the air. Nurses are expanding roles, gaining skills, and partnering with other health care providers to save lives and improve the health of all they serve.

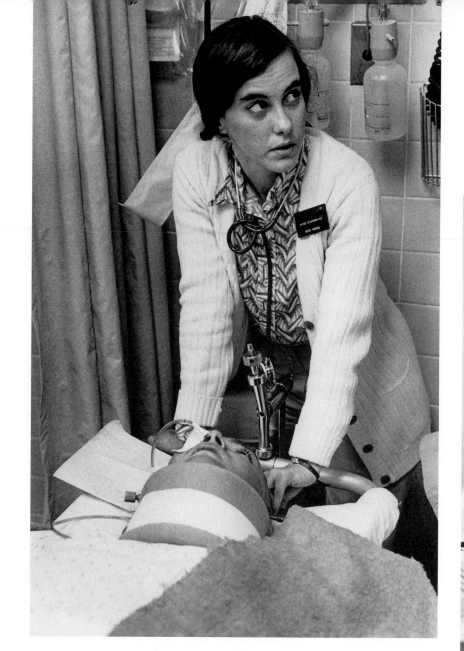

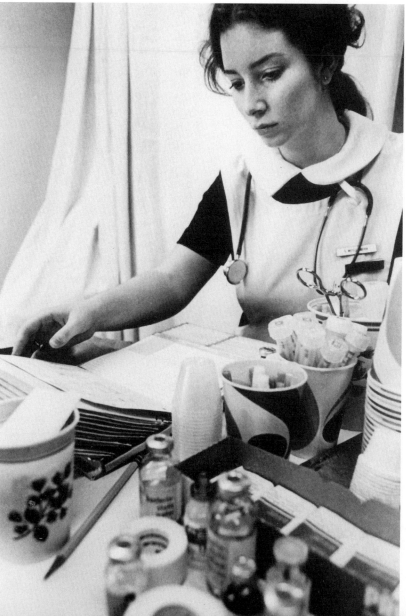

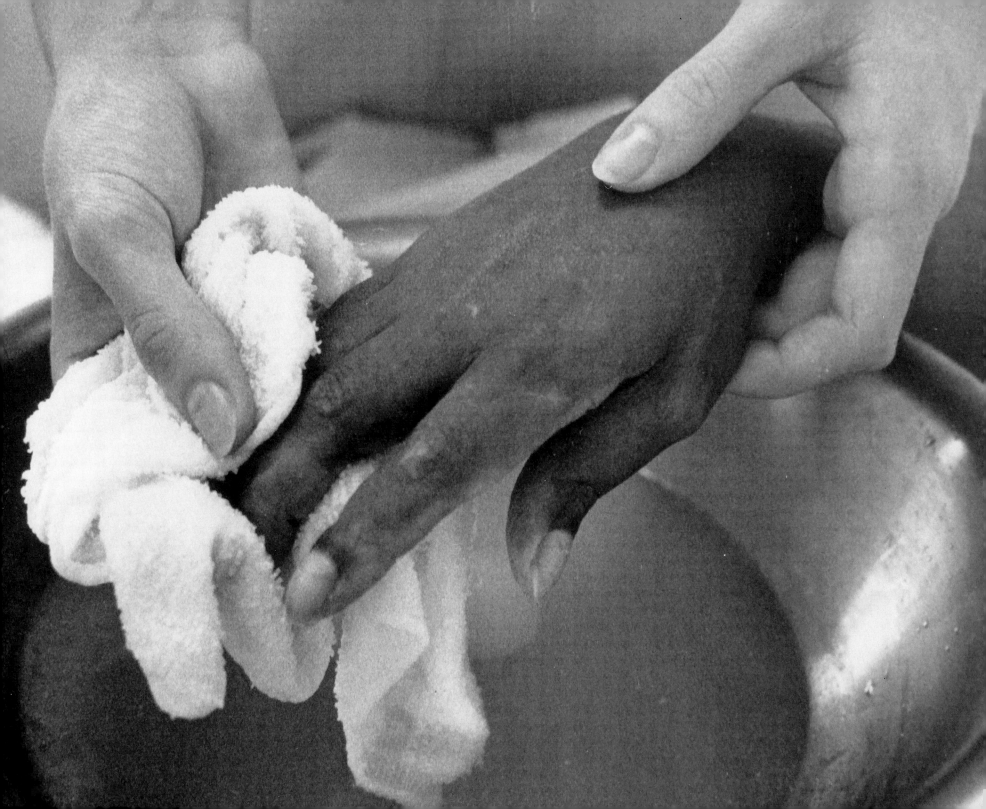

Nursing has given me the privilege of being with patients and families during times of vulnerability as well as times of great joy. As a hospital nurse, a public health nurse for Native Americans in the Southwest, and a family nurse practitioner in an urban area, I have come to appreciate the common desires and fears that unite all people. I have been humbled and at times, overwhelmed by the trust that patients place in me. At the same time, I have been energized by the possibility of making a difference in someone's life. No where is this more evident then in my role as a family nurse practitioner. Twenty-five years ago I was attracted to the nurse practitioner role because it offered me more autonomy in order to improve patient care.

Pioneering the NP role has been the most exhilarating part of my nursing career. I was challenged intellectually as I added new knowledge to my nursing base. I learned what it took to be a change agent, especially in some environments where change was not welcome. I was challenged as never before to articulate nursing's contribution to health care. Patients, communities, legislators, other professionals, and other nurses all questioned this new role. Responding to those questions was exciting, as that was an excellent opportunity to interpret the NP role and invite others to watch, listen, and experience my practice. Perhaps the greatest challenge of all was believing in myself as a primary care provider, that I was up to the task. I often felt the weight of the entire nurse practitioner movement on my shoulders.

Those early years felt like a proving ground where scrutiny and doubt were common. However, through the long hours, excessive learning, and critique by others, I was sustained by the positive response of patients and families. Patient acceptance came quickly, and I cherished the intimacy I developed with them over time. Patients knew that I could deliver effective care, listen and mutually plan with them, and refer if needed. I have loved every minute of being a nurse first and eventually a nurse practitioner.

Mary Ann Draye
SEATTLE, WASHINGTON

115

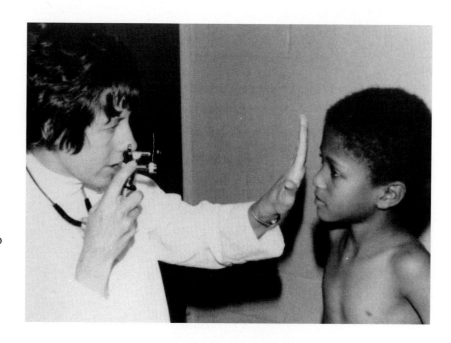

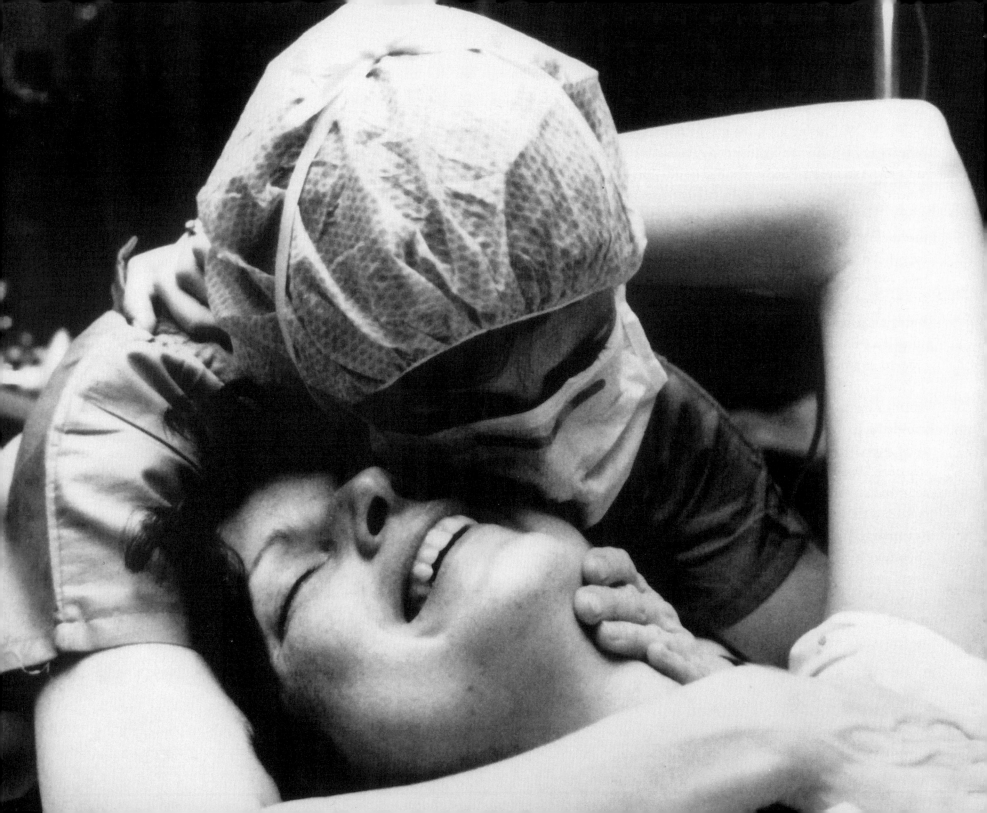

1980

Baby Fae, born with hypoplastic left heart syndrome, becomes the first newborn recipient of a cross-species heart transplant when she receives a baboon heart.

The United States leads a 58-nation boycott of the Moscow Olympics to protest the Soviet invasion of Afghanistan.

Inflation is running in the double digits, and gas costs around $1.20 a gallon.

Ex-Beatle John Lennon is fatally shot.

In Washington, Mount St. Helens erupts, producing an ash column more than 12 miles high.

Cigarette sales exceed $600 billion.

1981

The first cases of AIDS are identified in a small population of homosexual men in Los Angeles; a total of 422 cases are diagnosed in the United States.

Kaposi's sarcoma is first associated with HIV infection.

After 444 days in captivity, the American hostages in Iran are released as Ronald Reagan takes the presidential oath of office.

IBM introduces its personal computer.

Prince Charles of England marries Lady Diana Spencer.

Pope John Paul II and President Reagan are wounded in assassination attempts.

Sandra Day O'Connor becomes the first woman appointed to the Supreme Court.

1982

After implantation of the Jarvik-7 artificial heart, the recipient, Barney Clark, survives for 112 days.

The Food and Drug Administration approves human insulin produced in bacteria.

The Vietnam War Memorial is dedicated in Washington, D.C.

Johnson & Johnson pulls Tylenol capsules off the shelf after seven people die of cyanide poisoning caused by product tampering.

Compact discs become commercially available.

1983

The agent responsible AIDS, HIV, is isolated.

Microsoft releases Windows.

Cabbage Patch dolls become a fanatically sought item at Christmas.

1984

Crack cocaine is developed.

One sixth of Ethiopia's people are at risk of starvation during a famine.

The Internet opens to public use.

Apple Computer releases the first Macintosh personal computer.

1985

The FDA approves the first enzyme-linked immunosorbent assay (ELISA) test kit to screen for antibodies to HIV.

Mikhail Gorbachev comes to power in the Soviet Union and launches economic reforms and policies such as "glasnost" (openness), leading to a major easing of the Cold War.

1986

The Food and Drug Administration approves AZT, the first drug authorized for the treatment of AIDS.

The space shuttle Challenger explodes 13 seconds after liftoff, killing its seven-member crew, including Christa McAuliffe, a high-school teacher and the first private citizen to fly on the shuttle.

The world's worst nuclear incident, the Chernobyl meltdown, pollutes the environment and kills thousands.

1987

Ronald Reagan and Mikhail Gorbachev sign the treaty on nuclear arms.

The world's population exceeds 5 billion.

1988

The School of Nursing at the University of California-San Francisco becomes the first in the United States to offer a graduate curriculum in AIDS.

Surgeon General C. Everett Koop sends guidelines for preventing AIDS transmission to every U.S. household; almost 107,000 cases are diagnosed in the United States.

1989

East Berliners pour through the Berlin Wall as the barriers between East and West Germany begin to fall, paving the way for reunification of the country.

The Chinese military kills hundreds and arrests thousands more in Tiananmen Square in Beijing when students protest, demanding democratic reforms.

117

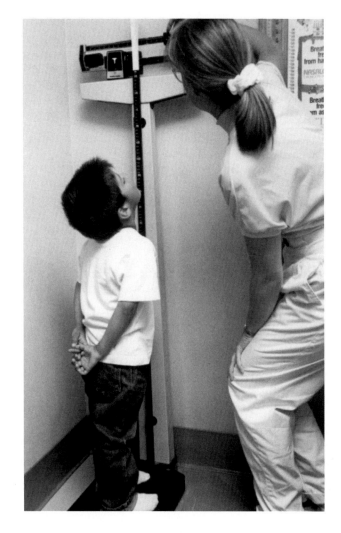

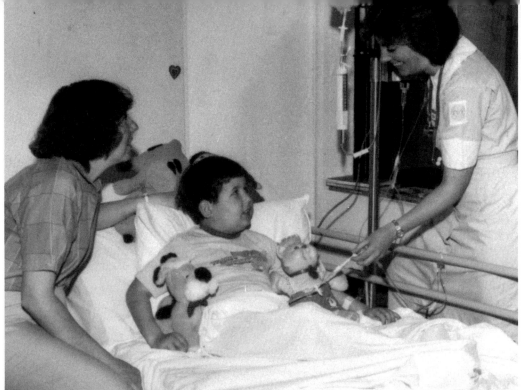

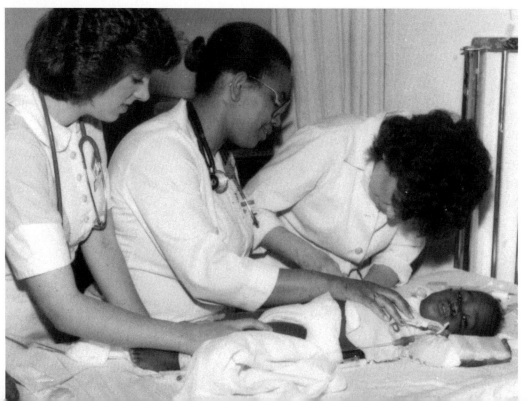

I was working as an emergency nurse practitioner in a free-standing emergency center located in a rural area. The unit was about 30 to 45 minutes from a hospital. Late in the afternoon, a mother and her son came into the unit. The mother seemed somewhat annoyed with her son but asked that I check him and tell him he was OK.

The history was that the patient had been working with his horse and the horse kicked him in the right upper quadrant of the abdomen about 2 hours previously and there had been pain in that area since then, which was getting worse. Upon getting him undressed, I saw a perfect bruise imprint of a horseshoe in the right upper quadrant extending onto the right lower rib area. The patient did not appear to be in any distress other than the pain in this area. He was not short of breath, orthostatic, or showing any signs that anything other than the bruise was wrong. However, when I tried to palpate the area, I was unable to get my fingers even slightly into the abdomen and nowhere close to the liver. This seemed to really increase his pain, and I began to worry about a liver injury.

I placed two large-bore IVs and called for the ambulance crew to prepare to transport him to the hospital. At this point, his mother told me that she could transport him in her car. I tried to explain that this was not a good idea and finally had to tell her that his life was in danger and she could not transport him in her car. She was extremely angry with me and let me know that she would speak to my supervisor. I told her that she was welcome to do that and gave her the name and number. In the meantime, her son was being transported to the hospital via ambulance.

I called the hospital ER and spoke with the doctor on duty and told him I thought the patient minimally needed a surgeon ASAP and probably the OR. The ER doc knew that I wasn't one to cry wolf and so he put out a stat call to the surgeon. This was before the days of trauma centers. The surgeon was in the ER when the patient arrived. The patient had started to become tachycardic and was showing signs of shock in the last 7 to 10 minutes of transport. He was taken immediately to the OR, where he was found to have a stellate fracture of the liver. This was repaired, and after multiple units of blood, he did very well.

I was working a 24-hour shift and did not get off until 10 AM the next morning. As I was finishing getting things ready for the change of shift, the mother of the patient came into the unit. She looked somewhat sheepish, and she said she thought she owed me an apology for the previous day and her behavior regarding her son. I told her that I knew he was okay now and that she was his mom and moms can't always be objective in these situations. She gave me a hug and thanked me for saving her son's life.

Linda L. Larson
LITTLETON, COLORADO

119

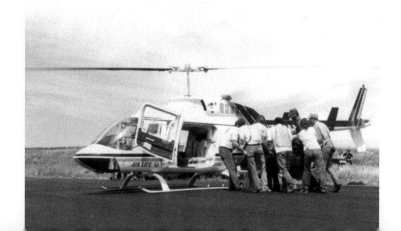

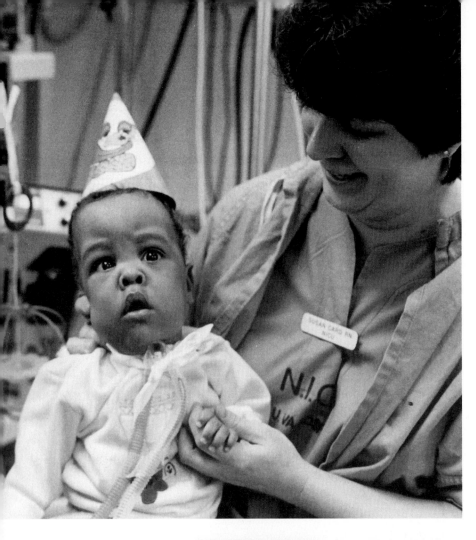

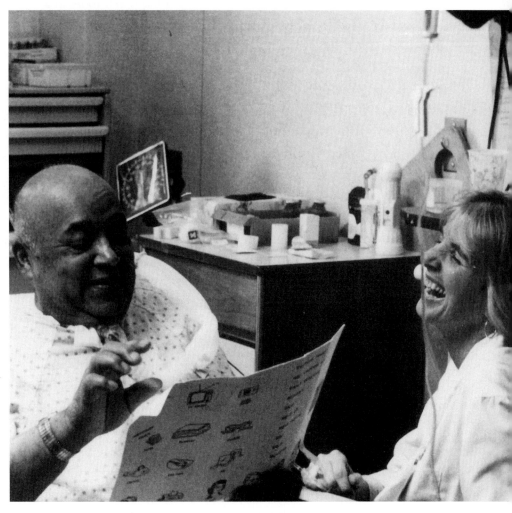

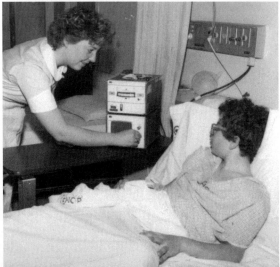

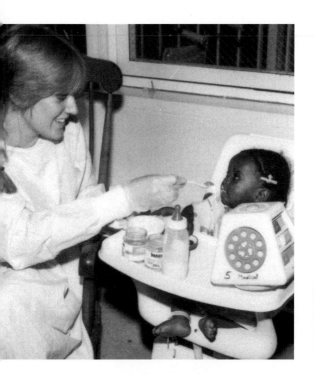

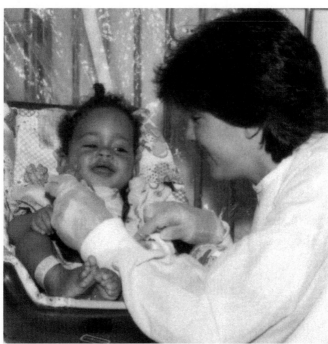

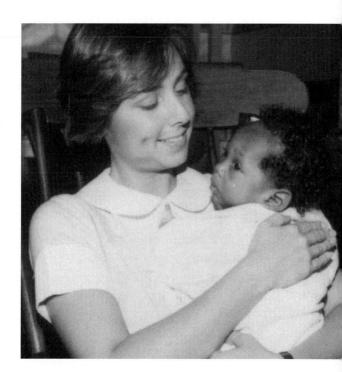

"*I*'d like a place of my own," was Nettie's answer to my question: "What can I help you with?" Nettie was one of my clients on my community treatment team. The team was her support, and we were charged with keeping individuals such as Nettie out of the State Mental Hospital that had housed her most of her adult life. I was to teach her independent living skills and to provide ongoing support and guidance.

Nettie was 84 years old, and it had been years since she had a place of her own. In her younger years, she had been married and had worked on a farm with her husband. She had a hard life during that time, with periodic interruptions where she was sent off to the psychiatric hospital for weeks, months, and even years.

I had my doubts from the start about her request to live alone. Nettie, on the other hand, knew I was a nurse and was confident that I would be able to help her for once and all live independently. With continuous trepidation, I worked right beside Nettie, and soon we were able to find her an apartment next to an assisted-living facility. She was thrilled, and I was proclaimed a true "angel of mercy." Each day Nettie would go to the senior center, and each evening she would be home just in time to meet the Meals-on-Wheels delivery volunteer. I would take her shopping each week, and when she wasn't looking, I would sneak in a little nursing assessment and medication check. She was able to live independently for almost 3 years before her elderly condition forced her into a nursing home closer to her sister and family.

Once she was provided with the opportunity to live outside the walls of the state institution, Nettie was able to see and believe in her own dream—all she needed from me was a little assistance. From my years of working with Nettie I learned that dreams can happen and that age is not important. Nettie taught me that change can happen and that having faith, patience, and persistence is important.

During my many years in nursing, I have worked with many wonderful people—but Nettie was special. From the first time I met her I knew she was someone who was holding on to her dreams. All she needed was a little opportunity and support. I am forever grateful that I was able to enrich Nettie's life, and equally important is how much she enriched mine.

Linda A. Bowers
WINTER GARDEN, FLORIDA

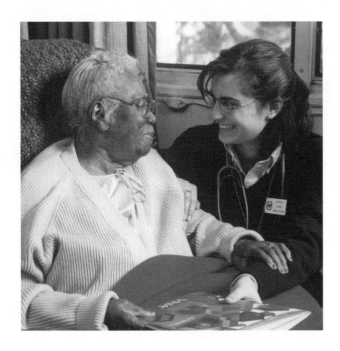

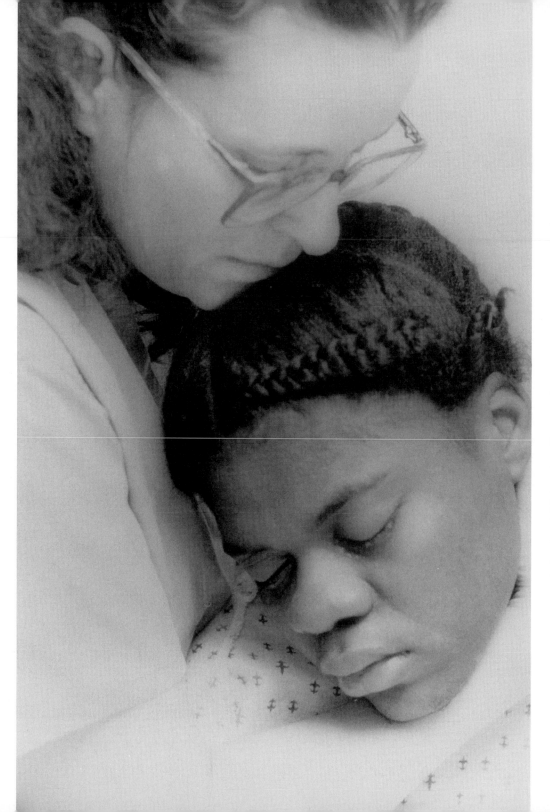

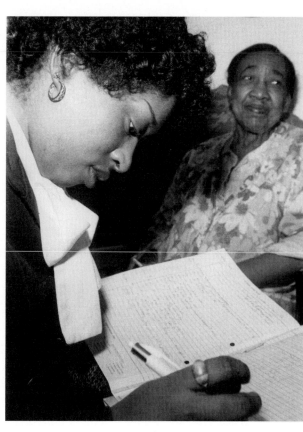

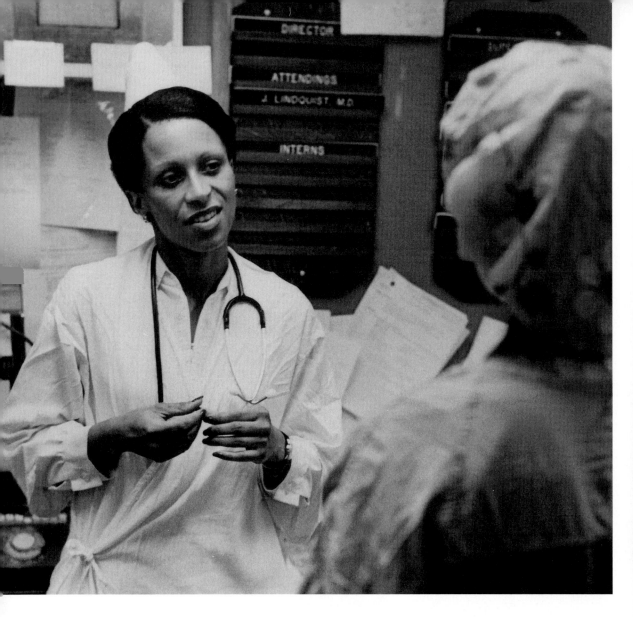
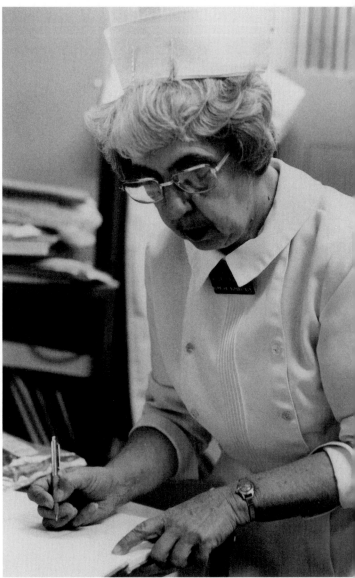

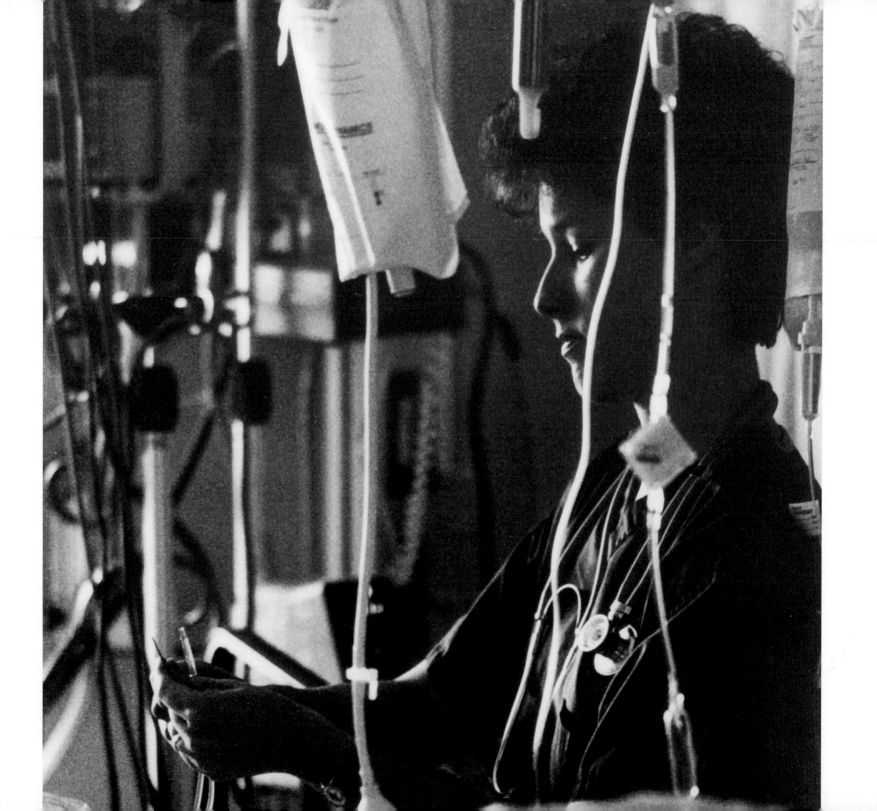

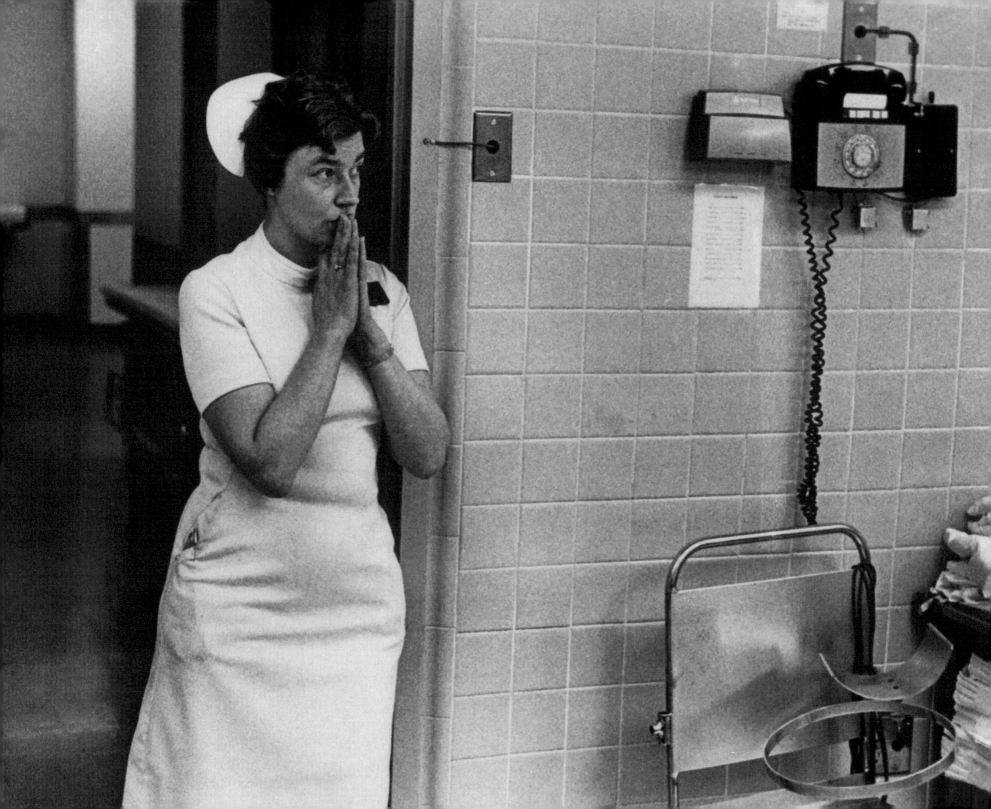

I'm not sure when the idea that I wanted to be a nurse first took root within me. After all, I was a grown woman with a family, and I thought that my course in life had already been set. Little did I know that nursing would become as firmly a part of me as would my two children.

The idea of becoming a nurse became imbedded in my conscious state at about the same time I first learned that I was pregnant. As the small embryo that was to become my daughter grew and formed, so did my desire to enter the profession of nursing. My swelling body and my unborn baby fascinated me, and I was hungry for information about what was happening to us. The lay books and pamphlets I had been reading did not tell me enough about this miracle called pregnancy, and my physician could not seem to provide me with the in-depth knowledge that I asked for.

Thus my friend Beth, a nurse, became my mentor and guide as she led me through the wonders of pregnancy. Beth loaned me her obstetric nursing textbooks and helped me satisfy my cravings for learning. Beth not only taught me about *pregnancy*, childbirth, and breastfeeding, she also taught me about the profession of nursing. I yearned to have her considerable knowledge, caring, and professional skills but never considered that nursing might be in my future.

By the time my son was born several years later, however, I was certain that I wanted to be a nurse. I again immersed myself in reading nursing textbooks and studied firsthand the caring professionalism of the nurses who helped my family and me during and after pregnancy. The birth of my second child, however, cinched the deal. Freshly home from the hospital with my newborn son at my breast and my 2-year-old daughter nestled close by, I dialed the local schools of nursing to find out what I needed to do.

The years have rolled by. My babies are now young adults, and I have been a nurse for more than 20 years. My children and my profession have thrived side by side, one complementing the other in ways that I could not have imagined. I look back on those days of learning and nurturing and growing with fondness and pride, and I feel fortunate for all that life has granted to me. Fully mature, my children continue to give meaning to my life and to fill my soul with purpose and joy, as does my chosen profession of nursing.

Pamela Meredith
ARLINGTON, VIRGINIA

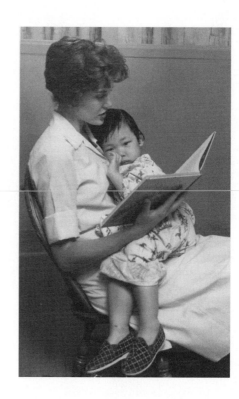

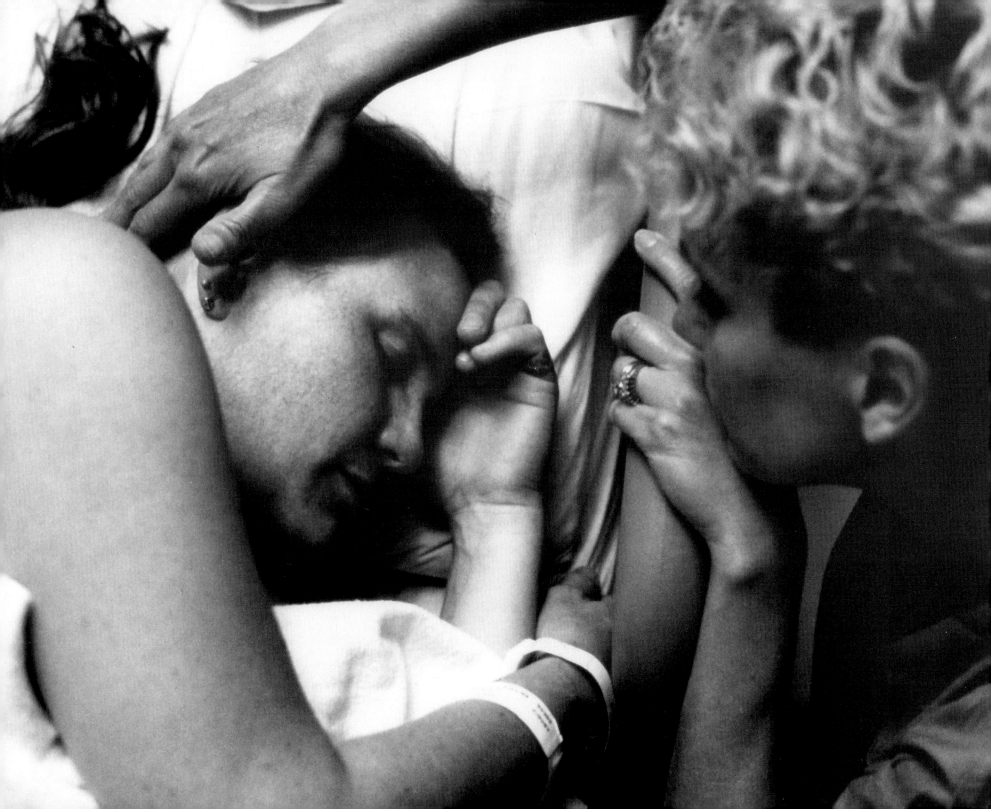

1990

The Human Genome Project begins.

The Hubble Space Telescope is deployed in low-Earth orbit (600 km).

L. Douglas Wilder is the first African-American man to be elected governor of a state (Virginia).

1991

The Baltic States regain their independence.

Operation Desert Storm ousts Iraqi troops from Kuwait.

A 5000-year-old body is found in the Austro-Italian Alps by mountain climbers.

The Soviet Union collapses, and Boris Yeltsin is inaugurated as the first freely elected president of the Russian Republic.

After a 70-year absence from the Western Hemisphere, cholera hits Peru and spreads to Brazil.

1992

Bosnia and Herzegovina secede from Yugoslavia.

A menopausal 53-year-old California woman gives birth to twins after in vitro fertilization using eggs from a donor and sperm from her husband.

The Food and Drug Administration restricts the use of silicone breast implants.

At midnight on December 31, Czechoslovakia is formally dissolved.

1993

A bomb explodes in the World Trade Center building, killing five people.

The Centers for Disease Control and Prevention identifies a new strain of the hantavirus, spread by deer mice in New Mexico.

1994

Jacqueline Bouvier Kennedy Onassis dies.

Nelson Mandela becomes the first black president of South Africa.

Hard-line Hutus slaughter or displace at least 3 million Tutsis.

1995

An outbreak of the killer Ebola virus occurs in Zaire, and Central and South America combat a major epidemic of dengue hemorrhagic fever.

On April 19, a truck parked outside the Alfred P. Murrah Federal Building in Oklahoma City explodes, killing 168 people dead, including 19 children.

A nerve gas attack in a Tokyo subway kills eight and injures thousands.

The Citadel in Charleston, South Carolina, announces that it will admit females.

1996

A possible link between "mad cow disease" in cattle and a new strain of the potentially fatal Creutzfeldt-Jakob disease in humans is reported.

Researchers develop a sensor that can detect E. coli.

Scientists predict global warming: a temperature rise of 1.8° to 6.3° F by 2100.

1997

A sheep, named Dolly, is successfully cloned in Edinburgh.

Researchers at the National Institutes of Health identify a gene abnormality that causes some cases of Parkinson's disease.

Diana, Princess of Wales, and Mother Teresa, leader of Missionaries of Charities, die.

Hong Kong is officially transferred to Chinese sovereignty.

The first set of live septuplets is born to an Iowa couple.

1998

Johns Hopkins University reports that an estimated 4 million Americans are infected with hepatitis C virus—about four times more than are infected with HIV.

The Centers for Disease Control and Prevention reports that HIV infection is no longer one of the top 10 killers in the United States.

American tobacco companies pay $206 million to settle lawsuits in 46 states.

President Clinton is impeached but does not leave office.

John Glenn, 77, becomes the oldest person to go into space.

The first step toward cloning a human is taken when an egg and a cell from an infertile woman are combined, creating a four-cell embryo.

1999

Two Columbine High School students shoot 12 fellow students and 1 teacher and wound another 23 before committing suicide.

The Dow Jones Industrial Average tops 10,000 for the first time and then tops 11,000 a month later.

The world population exceeds 6 billion.

Bertrand Piccard and Brian Jones become the first balloonists to circle the globe nonstop.

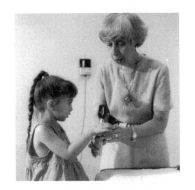

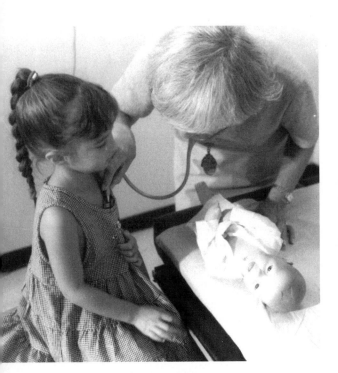

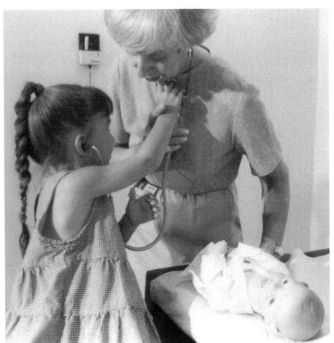

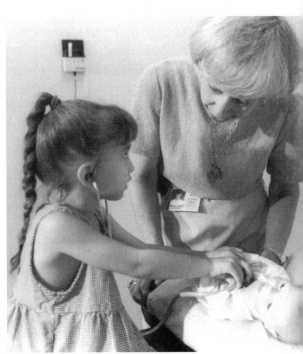

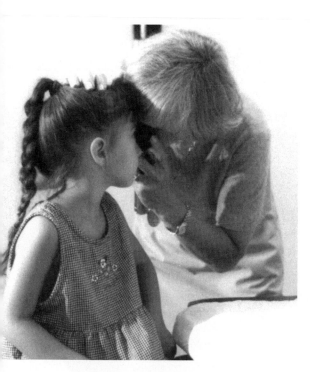

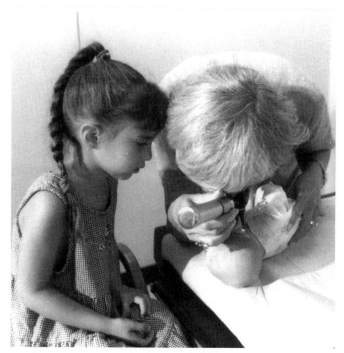

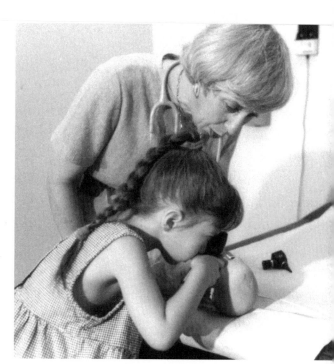

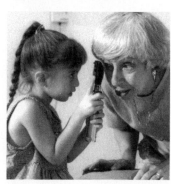

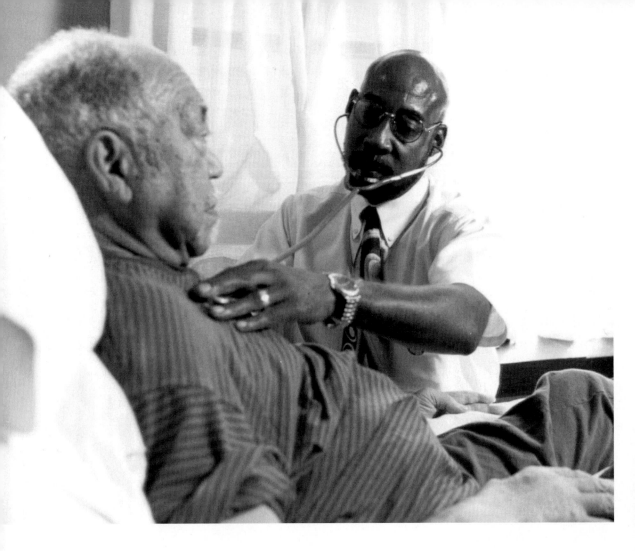

Nursing: A rich blend of knowledge, skill, caring, and technology.

My dad never had much in the way of a comfortable life. It was fraught with lack of money and learning to survive—often without a gentle hand or a kind word to guide him. His first young wife died leaving him with four daughters. He was not educated in the same sense that we know it. He remarried and had three more children, of whom I am the eldest. Though we were poor, he gave us a wealth unmatched by others in life, and death. When I saw you and your assistant bathing him so lovingly that last time, my heart was broken and joyous at the same time. Finally, although it was only minutes from his last breath, he was given a loving touch, a clean body, moist with lotion from your hands. My guess is it was the only time in his life that such a wonderful gift was given to him by anyone, including his own mother. With your help, he died peacefully, without pain, and with love.

A grateful daughter

133

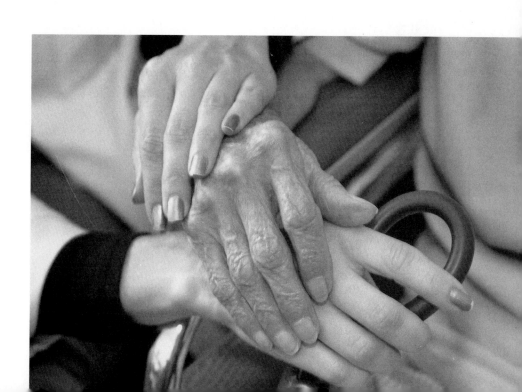

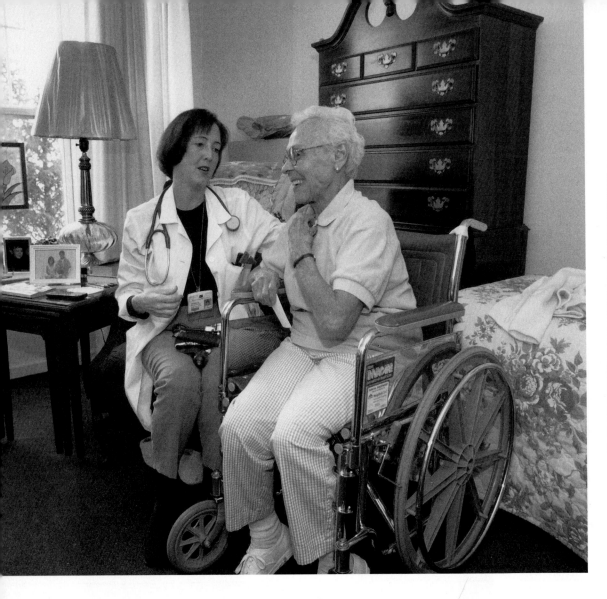

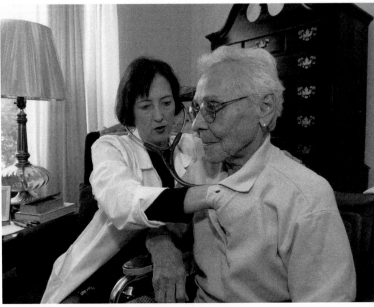

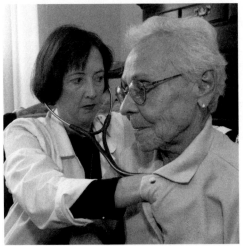

Helen, I know how hard you are working; you are making wonderful progress.

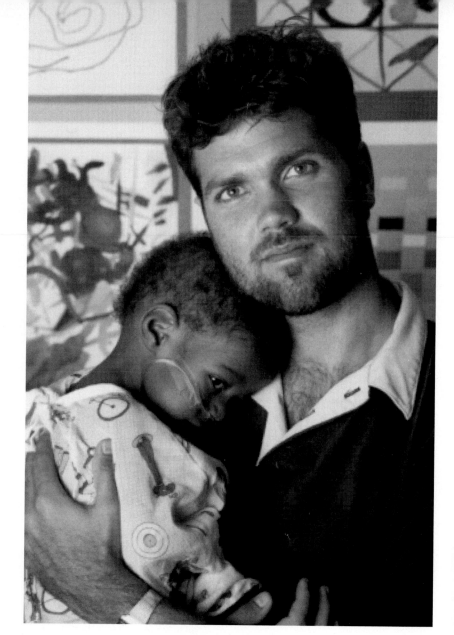

Georgia, a social worker, and I went together on a home visit to admit a patient to our hospice agency. An elderly brother and sister who had lived most of their lives together occupied the home. The patient was the elderly sister, and her brother was to be her caregiver. They had a number of cats as pets, and the cats obviously had the run of the house. After the admission visit, Georgia and I returned to our car. We started to feel itchy on our ankles and feet, and we soon realized that we both had been bitten by fleas. We wondered what to do to solve our problem, so we decided to purchase flea collars. The next visit, before we got out of the car, we slipped the flea collars onto our ankles and proceeded into the house. Success—the collars did the trick—no more bites. Later we will tackle ridding the house of the fleas.

A hospice nurse   135

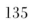

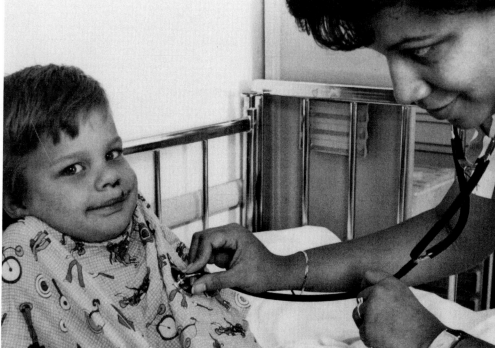

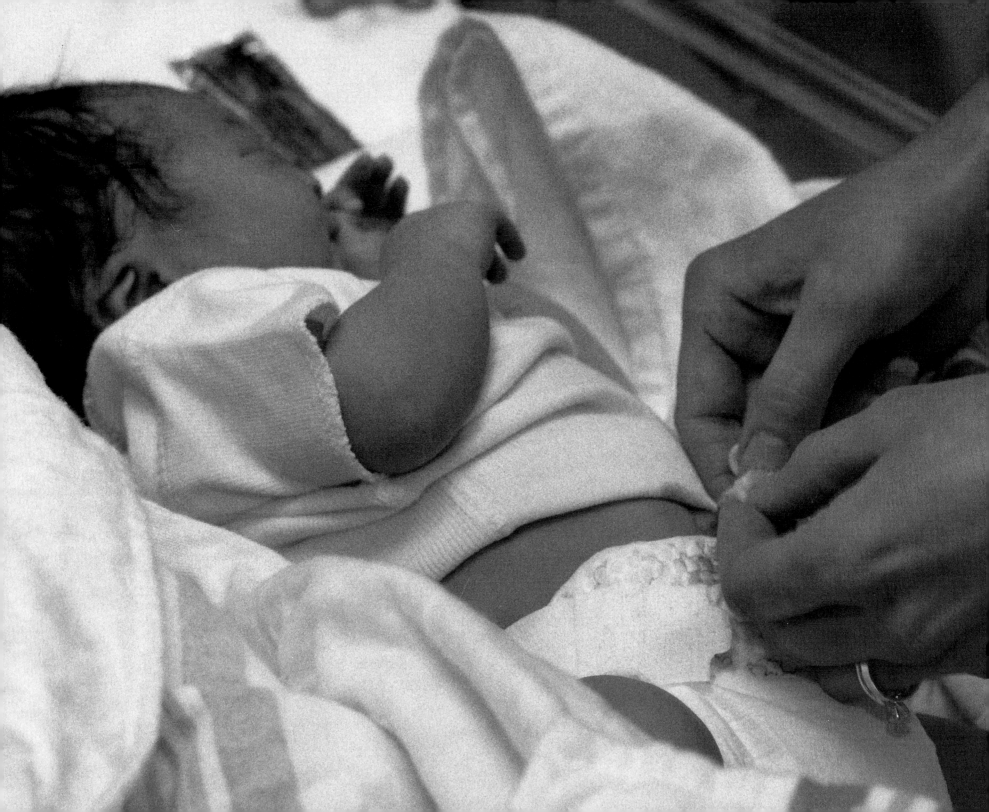

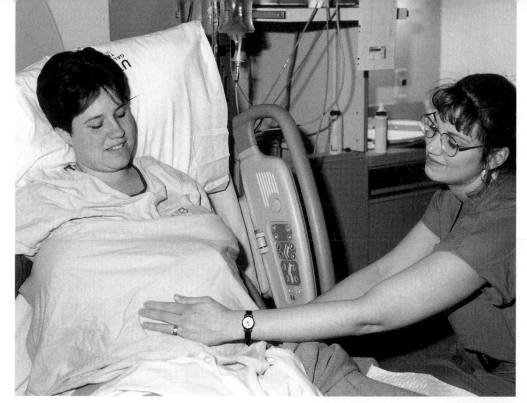

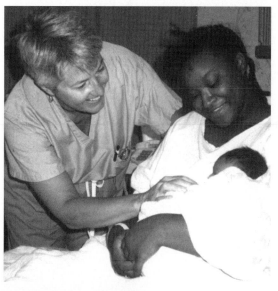

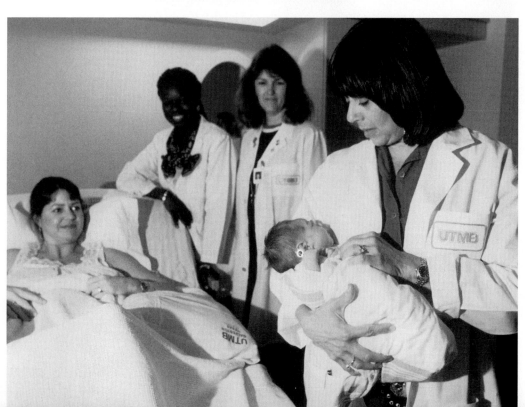

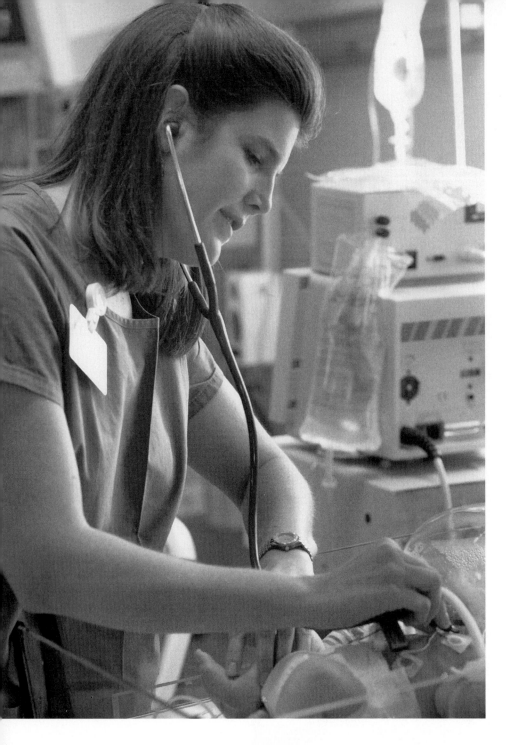

Nursing has been most rewarding for me as it has allowed me to assist others in their healing and/or dying process. The sick have taught me how to live, which helped me make informed choices or decisions later on. These experiences also helped me make lifestyle changes as well as take responsibility for my own health and life issues.

The highly sophisticated medical technology we have today need not intimidate one to neglect the important aspect of healing. To give oneself, to be present to another, to give of one's time is the greatest gift we can give another. Nursing has always challenged me in the giving of this gift.

Having kindness in my hands, in my eyes, in my heart, I will provide a loving, healing environment that may facilitate the healing of another. Love does such things as it brings transforming love to me and with all those with whom I come in contact with.

Sister Marie G. Frigo
Farmington, New Mexico

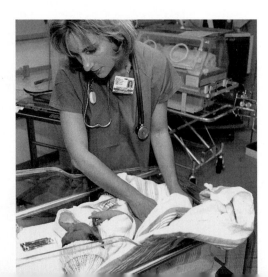

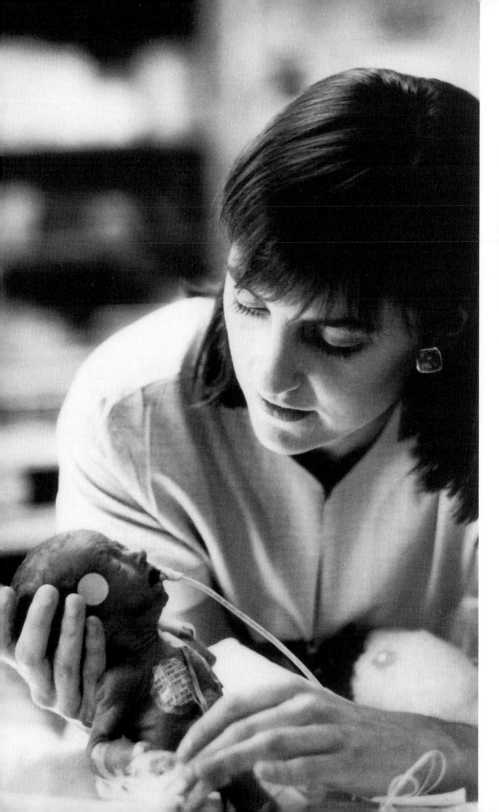

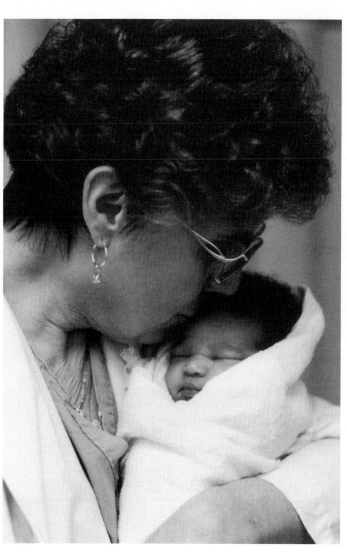

Precious care for precious gifts.

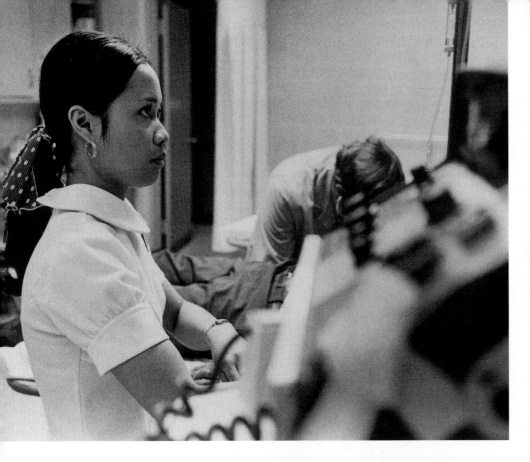
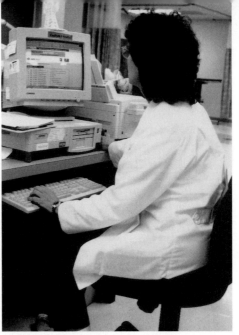
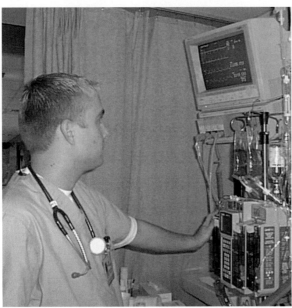
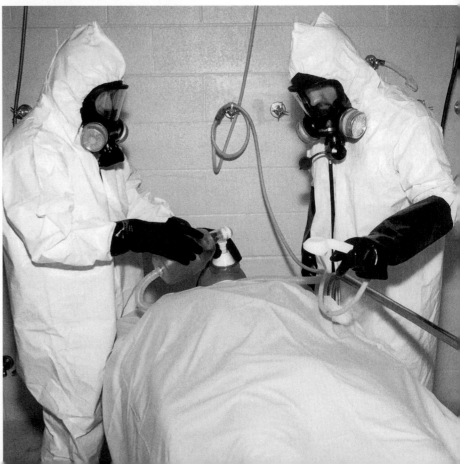

*Y*ou were there. You saw what I saw. You empathized and gave me the courage to face his deterioration and ultimate death. And, you did it with so much compassion. I had fears I had never felt before. And I wasn't sure I could hold on to my strength I needed for my sister, my mother, my brother, my father, and me. With a gentle firmness, you guided me—even in the middle of the night when his death was so very close. My exhaustion nearly got to me. I didn't think I could go on myself. But then, there you were again, with your encouraging words, your kindness, your understanding in the very height of my own sorrow.

The family member

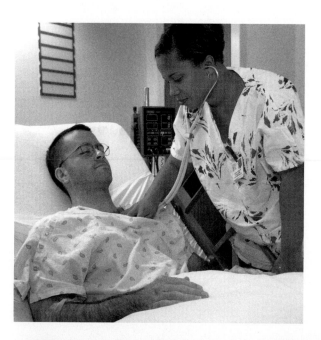

141

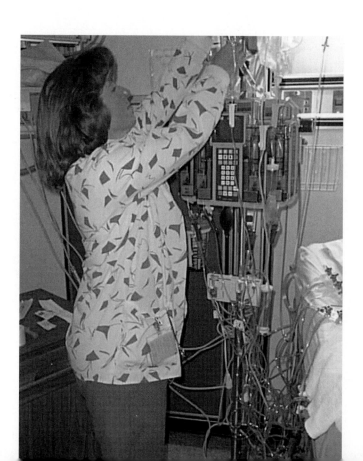

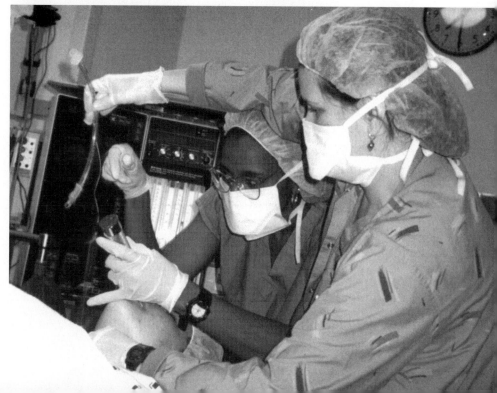

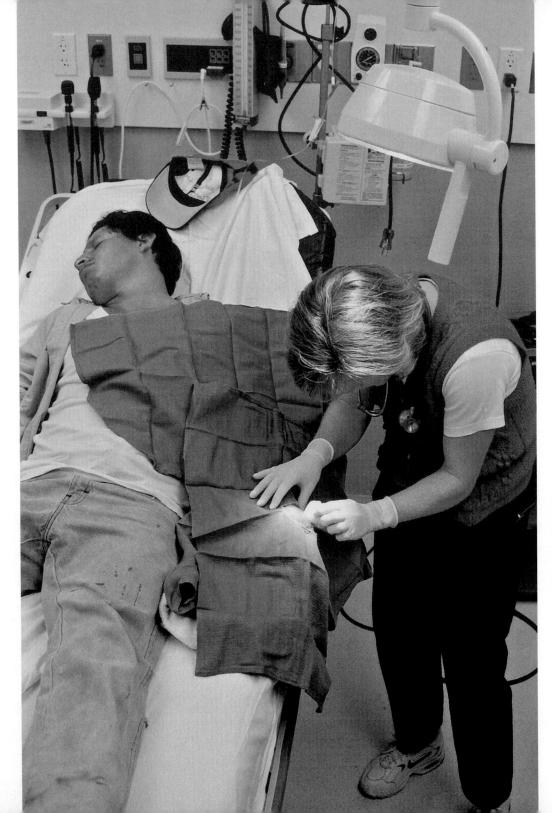

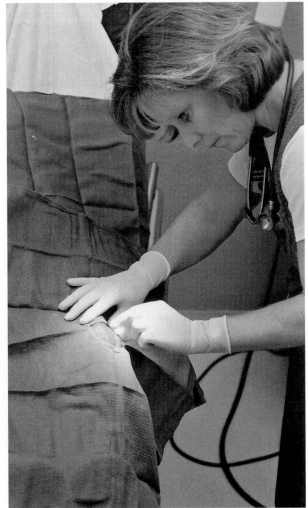

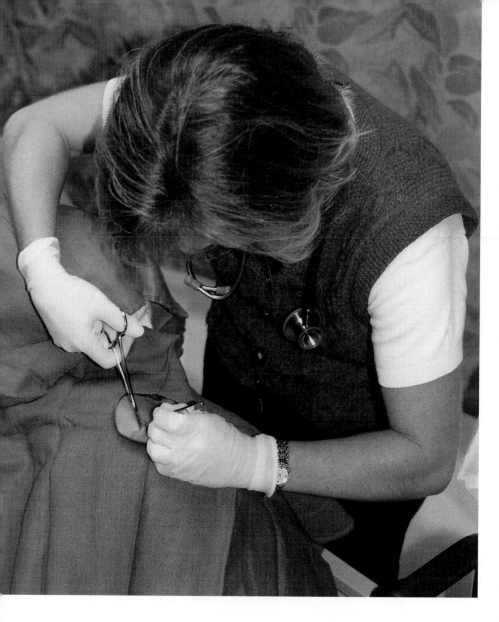

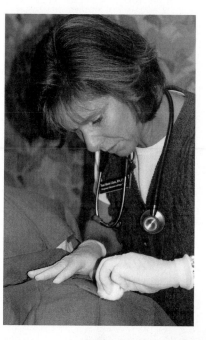

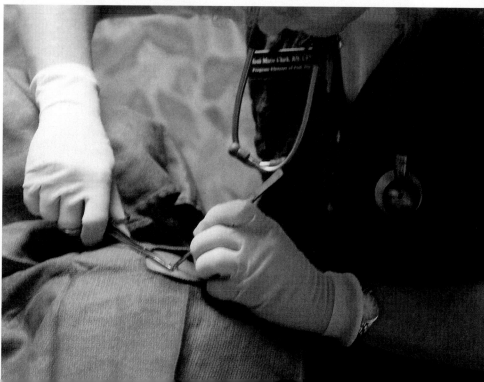

Nurse practitioners continue to expand the scope of nursing.

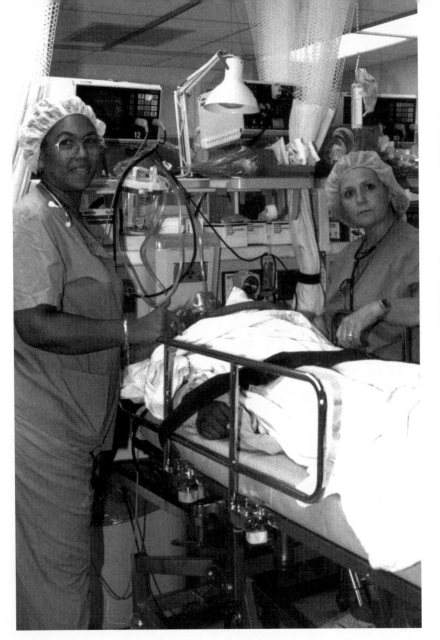

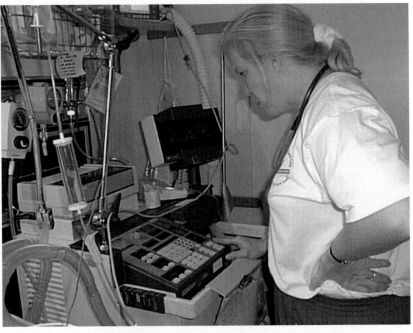

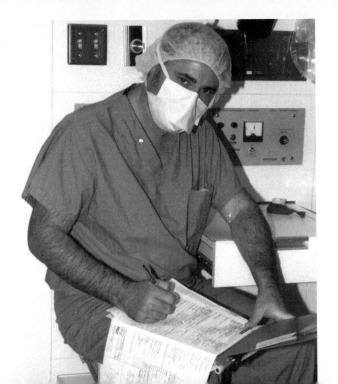

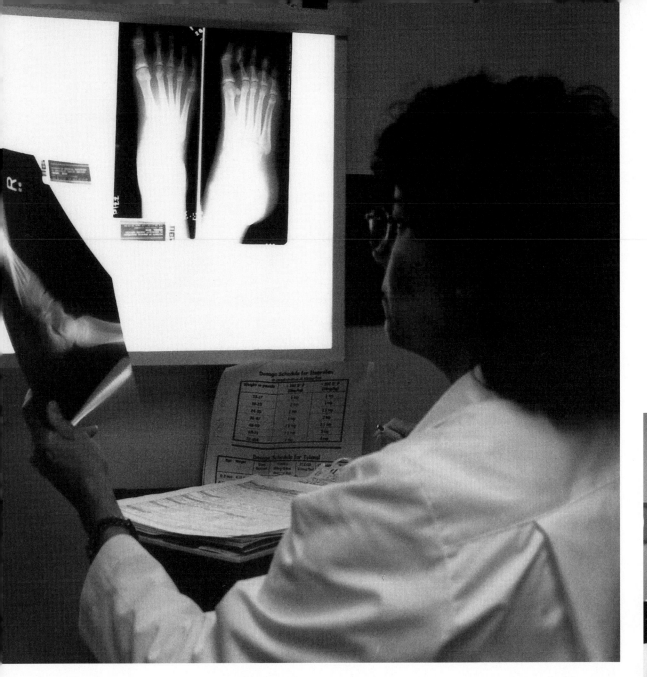

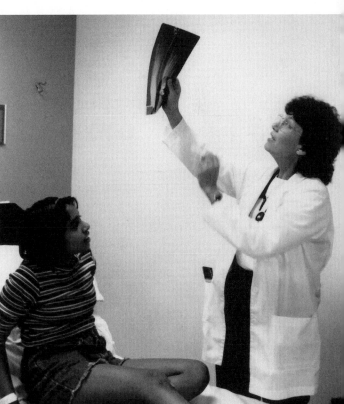

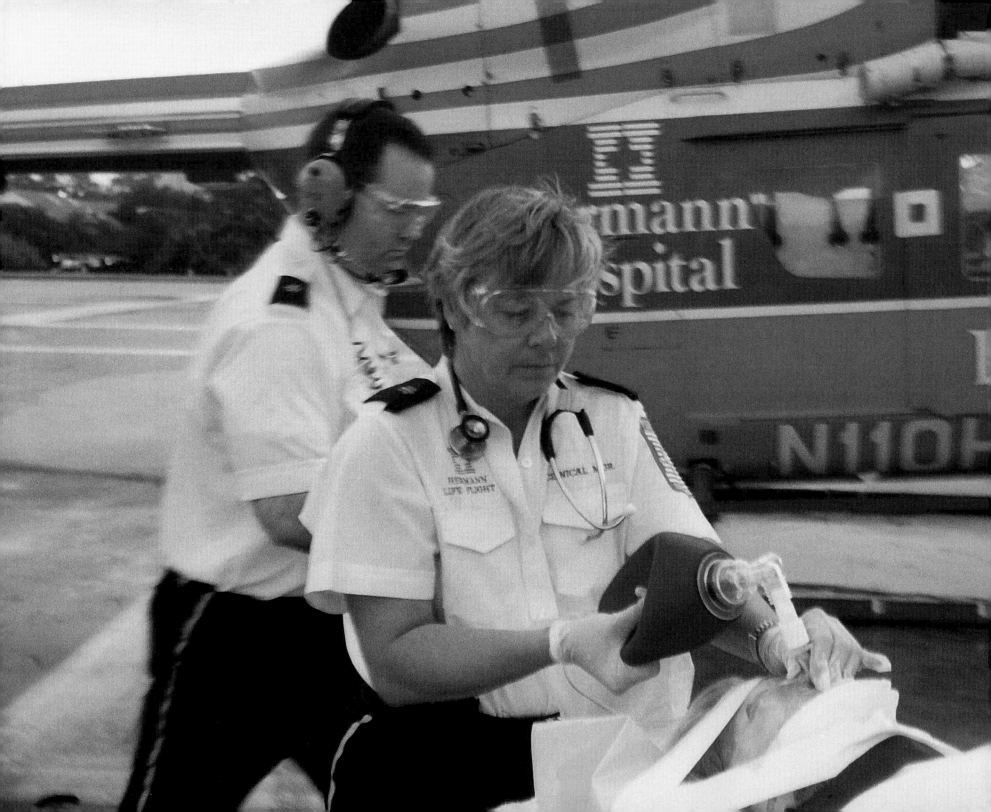

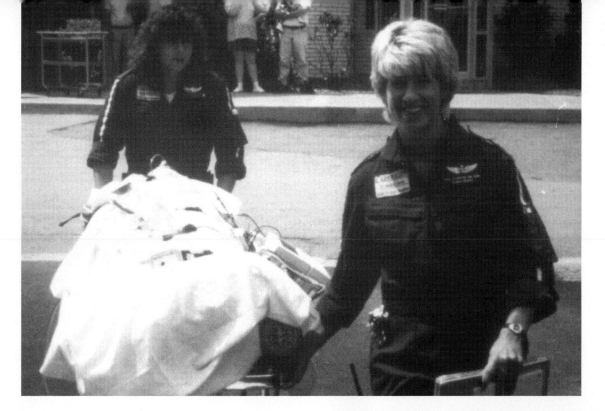

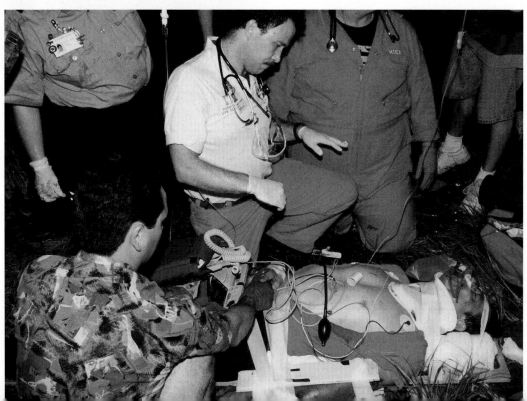

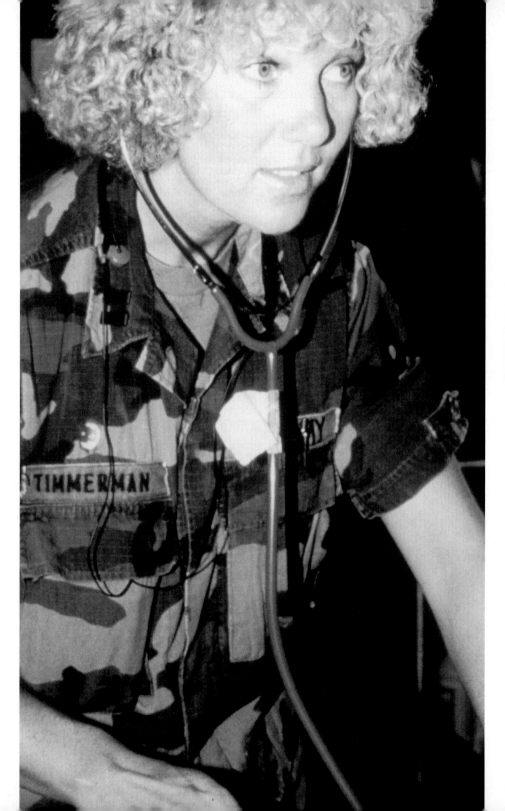

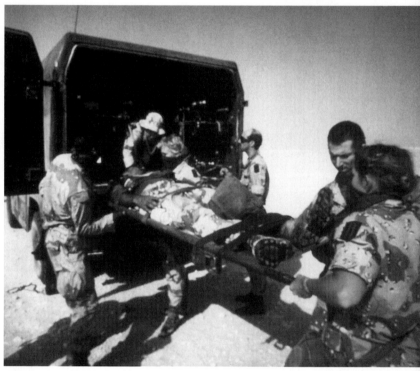

Operation Desert Storm.

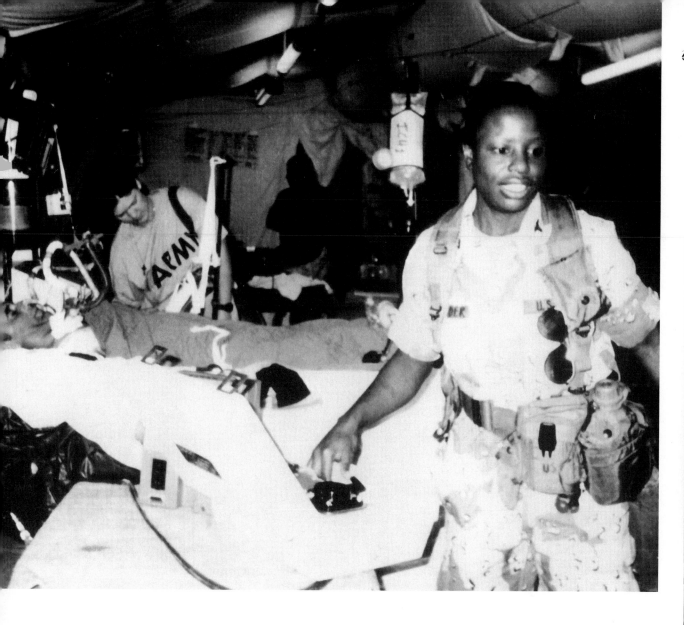

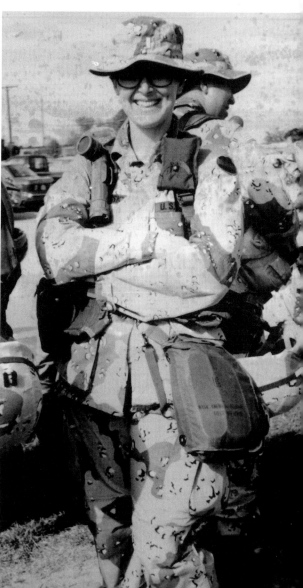

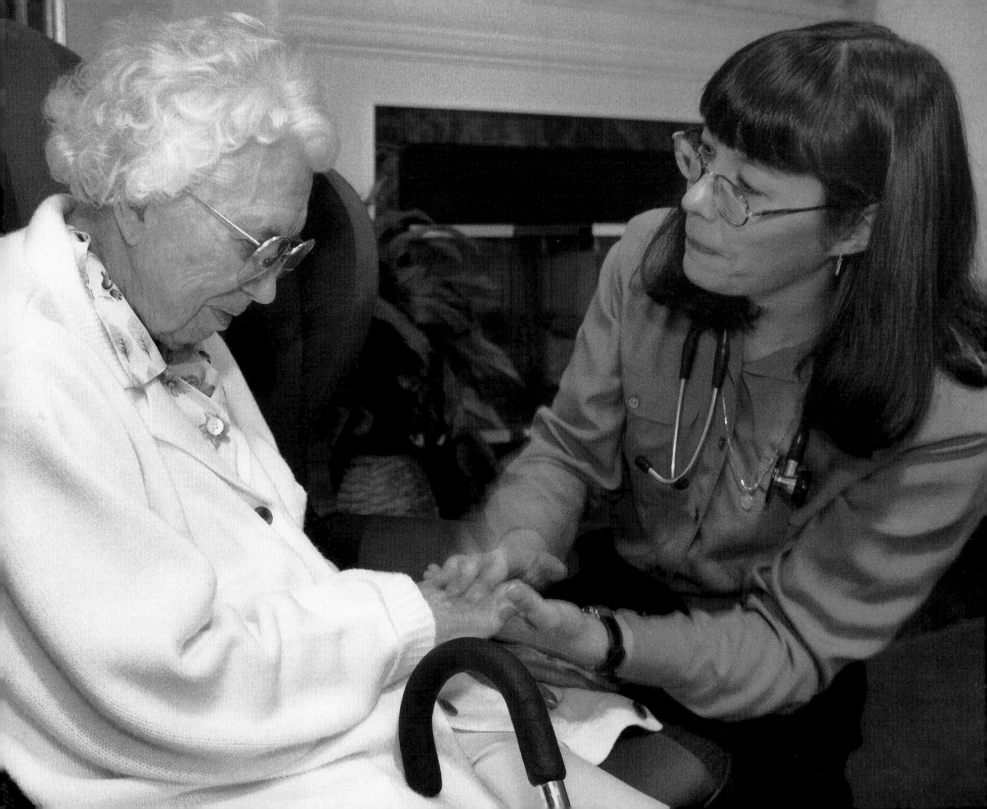

*E*very nurse knows the feeling, the role. Someone in the family is sick. They ask for advice in person or call halfway across the country. "What does it mean?" they ask. "What do you think?" "What should we do?" They seek out the nurse in the family.

This was my role during my mother's final years: case manager, health care system navigator, advocate, educator, coach, and through it all, her only daughter, her youngest child, her "Babe." It was a long road filled with hazards and challenges: fractured hip, rehab, wound infection, stroke, rehab, convalescence, assisted living, esophageal cancer, ICU, respiratory failure, and the end.

At the appointed time, we gathered. My two brothers and I waited in her room. The pulmonologist arrived, introduced himself, and shook everyone's hand. Standing close to my mother, and looking into her eyes, he spoke slowly. He explained the condition of her lungs, her options, and how he would help. With patience and grace he answered all questions, gave us his home phone number, and left. When the surgeon arrived, he stood at the foot of the bed and spoke to no one in particular. "Since the tube can't stay in any longer without causing damage, she needs to have a trach. I can schedule it for Monday. Let the nurses know if you have any questions." And with that, he left.

The silence was deafening. All eyes were on me. Mom picked up her clipboard, looked at me, and wrote in the beautiful cursive of a retired teacher, "I'm not sure what they were saying." Twenty years of nursing experience flashed through my brain—and my gut. I was never so grateful to be a nurse. I took a deep breath and began. My goal was to give her the information she needed to make her own choice. When I finished, she picked up her pad and wrote, "I love you ALL! Take the tube out." She died peacefully 2 days later in an ICU-turned-hospice bed, supported by many wise and caring nurses.

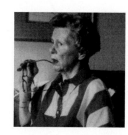

Mary Martha Hall
Houston, Texas

151

CREDITS

Front Matter

Postage stamps: Courtesy Dr. Pam Morgan, Houston, Texas.

1900-1909

p. xii: Courtesy Visiting Nurse Service of New York.

p. 3: From Armed Forces Institutes of Pathology.

p. 4, left: Courtesy Northwestern Memorial Hospital Archives, Chicago, Illinois.

p. 4, right: From Library of Congress.

p. 5, left: Courtesy Instructive Visiting Nurse Association of Richmond, Richmond, Virginia.

p. 5, right: From National Library of Medicine.

p. 7: Courtesy Rush-Presbyterian-St. Luke's Medical Center Archives, Chicago, Illinois.

1910-1919

p. 8: Courtesy MedStar Health Visiting Nurse Association serving Washington D.C., Maryland, and Northern Virginia.

p. 10, top: Courtesy MedStar Health Visiting Nurse Association serving Washington D.C., Maryland, and Northern Virginia.

p. 10, bottom: Courtesy MedStar Health Visiting Nurse Association serving Washington D.C., Maryland, and Northern Virginia.

p. 12, left: From Library of Congress.

p. 12, right: From Library of Congress.

p. 13, left: Courtesy Armed Forces Institutes of Pathology.

p. 13, right: From Library of Congress.

p. 14: From Library of Congress.

p. 16, left: From National Library of Medicine.

p. 16, right: Courtesy Instructive Visiting Nurse Association of Richmond, Richmond, Virginia.

p. 17, top: Courtesy National Library of Medicine.

p. 17, bottom: Courtesy Instructive Visiting Nurse Association of Richmond, Richmond, Virginia.

p. 18: From U.S. Army Military History Institute.

p. 19: From Library of Congress.

1920-1929

p. 20: From Library of Congress.

p. 22: From Library of Congress.

p. 23, upper left: Courtesy MedStar Health Visiting Nurse Association serving Washington D.C., Maryland, and Northern Virginia.

p. 23, lower left: Courtesy MedStar Health Visiting Nurse Association serving Washington D.C., Maryland, and Northern Virginia.

p. 23: upper right: Courtesy MedStar Health Visiting Nurse Association serving Washington D.C., Maryland, and Northern Virginia.

p. 23, lower right: Courtesy MedStar Health Visiting Nurse Association serving Washington D.C., Maryland, and Northern Virginia.

p. 24, left: Courtesy MedStar Health Visiting Nurse Association serving Washington D.C., Maryland, and Northern Virginia.

p. 24, upper right: Courtesy MedStar Health Visiting Nurse Association serving Washington D.C., Maryland, and Northern Virginia.

p. 24, lower right: Courtesy MedStar Health Visiting Nurse Association serving Washington D.C., Maryland, and Northern Virginia.

p. 25: Courtesy MedStar Health Visiting Nurse Association serving Washington D.C., Maryland, and Northern Virginia.

p. 27, top: From Library of Congress.

p. 27, bottom: Courtesy Center for Nursing Historical Inquiry, University of Virginia School of Nursing, Charlottesville, Virginia.

p. 28: Courtesy Center for Nursing Historical Inquiry, University of Virginia School of Nursing, Charlottesville, Virginia.

p. 29, top: Courtesy Center for Nursing Historical Inquiry, University of Virginia School of Nursing, Charlottesville, Virginia.

p. 29, bottom: Courtesy Center for Nursing Historical Inquiry, University of Virginia School of Nursing, Charlottesville, Virginia.

p. 30, top: Courtesy Visiting Nurse Association of Greater Philadelphia.

p. 30, *bottom:* Courtesy Center for Nursing Historical Inquiry, University of Virginia School of Nursing, Charlottesville, Virginia.

p. 31, *top:* From Library of Congress.

p. 31, *bottom:* From National Library of Medicine.

1930-1939

p. 32: From Library of Congress.

p. 34, *left:* From Library of Congress.

p. 34, *right:* Courtesy MedStar Health Visiting Nurse Association serving Washington D.C., Maryland, and Northern Virginia.

p. 35: Courtesy St. Vincent Health System, Little Rock, Arkansas.

p. 36, *top:* Courtesy MedStar Health Visiting Nurse Association serving Washington D.C., Maryland, and Northern Virginia.

p. 36, *bottom:* Courtesy MedStar Health Visiting Nurse Association serving Washington D.C., Maryland, and Northern Virginia.

p. 37: Courtesy Northwestern Memorial Hospital Archives, Chicago, Illinois.

p. 38: From Library of Congress.

p. 39, *top:* From Library of Congress.

p. 39, *bottom:* Courtesy Frontier Nursing Service, Wendover, Kentucky.

p. 40, *left:* Courtesy Visiting Nurse Association of Greater Philadelphia.

p. 40, *right:* Courtesy MedStar Health Visiting Nurse Association serving Washington D.C., Maryland, and Northern Virginia.

p. 41, *top:* From Library of Congress.

p. 41, *lower left:* From Library of Congress.

p. 41, *lower right:* From Library of Congress.

p. 42: Courtesy Instructive Visiting Nurse Association of Richmond, Richmond, Virginia.

p. 43: Courtesy Frontier Nursing Service, Wendover, Kentucky.

p. 44, *left:* Courtesy Frontier Nursing Service, Wendover, Kentucky.

p. 44, *upper right:* From National Library of Medicine.

p. 44, *lower right:* Courtesy Frontier Nursing Service, Wendover, Kentucky.

p. 45: Courtesy Frontier Nursing Service, Wendover, Kentucky.

1940-1949

p. 46: From National Archives and Records Administration.

p. 48, *upper left:* From Library of Congress.

p. 48, *lower left:* From Library of Congress.

p. 48, *lower middle:* From Library of Congress.

p. 48, *right:* From National Library of Medicine.

p. 49, *upper left:* From Library of Congress.

p. 49, *middle:* From Library of Congress.

p. 49, *upper middle:* From Library of Congress.

p. 49, *lower left:* From National Library of Medicine.

p. 49, *right:* From National Archives and Records Administration.

p. 50: From Library of Congress.

p. 51, *upper left:* Courtesy American Heritage Center, University of Wyoming, Laramie, Wyoming.

p. 51, *lower left:* From National Archives and Records Administration.

p. 51, *right:* Courtesy American Heritage Center, University of Wyoming, Laramie, Wyoming.

p. 52, *left:* From National Archives and Records Administration.

p. 52, *upper right:* From U.S. Army Center of Military History.

p. 52, *bottom middle:* From Library of Congress.

p. 52, *bottom right:* From Library of Congress.

p. 53, *left:* From National Archives and Records Administration.

p. 53, *right:* From National Archives and Records Administration.

p. 54: From National Library of Medicine.

p. 55, *top:* From National Archives and Records Administration.

p. 55, *bottom:* From National Library of Medicine.

p. 56: Courtesy American Heritage Center, University of Wyoming, Laramie, Wyoming.

154

p. 57: upper left: From National Library of Medicine.

p. 57, lower left: From Library of Congress.

p. 57, right: From Library of Congress.

p. 58: From U.S. Army Center of Military History.

p. 59, top: From Library of Congress.

p. 59, bottom: From Library of Congress.

p. 60, top: Courtesy Center for Nursing Historical Inquiry, University of Virginia School of Nursing, Charlottesville, Virginia.

p. 60, bottom: From Library of Congress.

p. 61, top: From Library of Congress.

p. 61, bottom: From Library of Congress.

p. 62, left: Courtesy Center for the Study of the History of Nursing, University of Pennsylvania School of Nursing, Philadelphia, Pennsylvania.

p. 62, right: Courtesy Center for the Study of the History of Nursing, University of Pennsylvania School of Nursing, Philadelphia, Pennsylvania.

p. 63, top: From Library of Congress.

p. 63, lower left: From Library of Congress.

p. 63, lower right: From National Library of Medicine.

p. 64, top: From Library of Congress.

p. 64, bottom: From National Library of Medicine.

p. 65: Courtesy Visiting Nurse Association of Greater Philadelphia.

p. 66: Library of Congress.

p. 67, top left: From National Library of Medicine.

p. 67, lower left: From Library of Congress.

p. 67, top right: From Library of Congress.

p. 67, lower right: From Library of Congress.

1950–1959

p. 68: Courtesy Visiting Nurse Association of Greater Philadelphia.

p. 70, top left: From National Archives and Records Administration.

p. 70, lower left: From U.S. Army Center of Military History.

p. 70, top right: From U.S. Army Center of Military History.

p. 70 lower right: From U.S. Army Center of Military History.

p. 71, top: Courtesy MedStar Health Visiting Nurse Association serving Washington D.C., Maryland, and Northern Virginia.

p. 71, bottom: Courtesy MedStar Health Visiting Nurse Association serving Washington D.C., Maryland, and Northern Virginia.

p. 72, top left: From Library of Congress.

p. 72, lower left: From Library of Congress.

p. 72, right: From Library of Congress.

p. 73: Courtesy Marian Louise Goff, Louisville, Kentucky.

p. 74, top: Courtesy Center for the Study of the History of Nursing, University of Pennsylvania School of Nursing, Philadelphia, Pennsylvania.

p. 74, lower left: Courtesy Center for Nursing Historical Inquiry, University of Virginia School of Nursing, Charlottesville, Virginia.

p. 74, lower right: Courtesy Center for Nursing Historical Inquiry, University of Virginia School of Nursing, Charlottesville, Virginia.

p. 75, left: From National Library of Medicine and World Health Organization.

p. 75, top middle: Courtesy Center for the Study of the History of Nursing, University of Pennsylvania School of Nursing, Philadelphia, Pennsylvania.

p. 75, center middle: Courtesy Northwestern Memorial Hospital Archives, Chicago, Illinois.

p. 75, lower middle: Courtesy Center for Nursing Historical Inquiry, University of Virginia School of Nursing, Charlottesville, Virginia.

p. 75, right: Courtesy Center for the Study of the History of Nursing, University of Pennsylvania School of Nursing, Philadelphia, Pennsylvania.

p. 76, top left: From Library of Congress.

p. 76, bottom left: Courtesy MedStar Health Visiting Nurse Association serving Washington D.C., Maryland, and Northern Virginia.

p. 76, top right: From Library of Congress.

p. 76, bottom right: Courtesy MedStar Health Visiting Nurse Association serving Washington D.C., Maryland, and Northern Virginia.

p. 77, top: Courtesy Marian Louise Goff, Louisville, Kentucky.

p. 77, lower left: From Library of Congress.

p. 77, lower middle: From Library of Congress.

p. 77: lower right: Courtesy Center for the Study of the History of Nursing, University of Pennsylvania School of Nursing, Philadelphia, Pennsylvania.

p. 78: Courtesy MedStar Health Visiting Nurse Association serving Washington D.C., Maryland, and Northern Virginia.

p. 79, left: Courtesy Visiting Nurse Association of Greater Philadelphia.

p. 79, top right: From National Library of Medicine and World Health Organization.

p. 79, lower right: From National Library of Medicine and World Health Organization.

p. 80, top left: Courtesy Visiting Nurse Association of Greater Philadelphia.

p. 80, lower left: Courtesy Center for the Study of the History of Nursing, University of Pennsylvania School of Nursing, Philadelphia, Pennsylvania.

p. 80, top right: From Library of Congress.

p. 80, lower right: From Library of Congress.

p. 81: From National Library of Medicine.

p. 82: From National Library of Medicine.

p. 83, top left: Courtesy MedStar Health Visiting Nurse Association serving Washington D.C., Maryland, and Northern Virginia.

p. 83, lower left: From Library of Congress.

p. 83, top right: Courtesy MedStar Health Visiting Nurse Association serving Washington D.C., Maryland, and Northern Virginia.

p. 83, lower right: From Library of Congress.

p. 84: From Library of Congress.

p. 85, top left: Courtesy MedStar Health Visiting Nurse Association serving Washington D.C., Maryland, and Northern Virginia.

p. 85: lower left: Courtesy MedStar Health Visiting Nurse Association serving Washington D.C., Maryland, and Northern Virginia.

p. 85, right: Courtesy Visiting Nurse Service of New York.

1960-1969

p. 86: Courtesy Visiting Nurse Association of Greater Philadelphia.

p. 88, left: Courtesy Northwestern Memorial Hospital Archives, Chicago, Illinois.

p. 88, top right: Courtesy Northwestern Memorial Hospital Archives, Chicago, Illinois.

p. 88, lower right: From Library of Congress.

p. 89, left: Courtesy Northwestern Memorial Hospital Archives, Chicago, Illinois.

p. 89, right: Courtesy Center for the Study of the History of Nursing, University of Pennsylvania School of Nursing, Philadelphia, Pennsylvania.

p. 90, left: From National Library of Medicine and World Health Organization.

p. 90, right: From National Library of Medicine and World Health Organization.

p. 91: From National Library of Medicine and World Health Organization.

p. 92: From Hampton University Archives, Hampton, Virginia.

p. 93, top left: Courtesy MedStar Health Visiting Nurse Association serving Washington D.C., Maryland, and Northern Virginia.

p. 93, top right: Courtesy MedStar Health Visiting Nurse Association serving Washington D.C., Maryland, and Northern Virginia.

p. 93, bottom: Courtesy Rush-Presbyterian-St. Luke's Medical Center Archives, Chicago, Illinois.

p. 94, left: Courtesy MedStar Health Visiting Nurse Association serving Washington D.C., Maryland, and Northern Virginia.

p. 94, center: Courtesy MedStar Health Visiting Nurse Association serving Washington D.C., Maryland, and Northern Virginia.

p. 94, right: Courtesy MedStar Health Visiting Nurse Association serving Washington D.C., Maryland, and Northern Virginia.

p. 95, left: Courtesy Center for Nursing Historical Inquiry, University of Virginia School of Nursing, Charlottesville, Virginia.

1980-1989

p. 116: Photograph by Harriette Hartigan, Ann Arbor, Michigan, website: www.harriettehartigan.com, e-mail: H2inA2@aol.com.

p. 118, left: Courtesy University of California-Los Angeles School of Nursing.

p. 118, top right: Courtesy Villanova University College of Nursing, Villanova, Pennsylvania.

p. 118, lower right: Courtesy Villanova University College of Nursing, Villanova, Pennsylvania.

p. 119: Courtesy Jill Johnson, Lexington, Kentucky.

p. 120, top left: Courtesy Center for Nursing Historical Inquiry, University of Virginia School of Nursing, Charlottesville, Virginia.

p. 120, lower left: Courtesy Villanova University College of Nursing, Villanova, Pennsylvania.

p. 120, right: Courtesy Center for Nursing Historical Inquiry, University of Virginia School of Nursing, Charlottesville, Virginia.

p. 121, left: Courtesy Villanova University College of Nursing, Villanova, Pennsylvania.

p. 121, center: Courtesy Villanova University School of Nursing, Villanova, Pennsylvania.

p. 121, right: Courtesy Villanova University School of Nursing, Villanova, Pennsylvania.

p. 122: Courtesy MedStar Health Visiting Nurse Association serving Washington D.C., Maryland, and Northern Virginia.

p. 123, left: Photograph by Harriette Hartigan, Ann Arbor, Michigan, website: www.harriettehartigan.com, e-mail: H2inA2@aol.com.

p. 123, right: Courtesy MedStar Health Visiting Nurse Association serving Washington D.C., Maryland, and Northern Virginia.

p. 124, left: Courtesy Northwestern Memorial Hospital Archives, Chicago, Illinois.

p. 124, right: Courtesy Northwestern Memorial Hospital Archives, Chicago, Illinois.

p. 125: Courtesy Center for Nursing Historical Inquiry, University of Virginia School of Nursing, Charlottesville, Virginia.

p. 126: Courtesy Northwestern Memorial Hospital Archives, Chicago, Illinois.

p. 127: Courtesy University of California-Los Angeles School of Nursing.

1990-1999

p. 128: Photograph by Harriette Hartigan, Ann Arbor, Michigan, website: www.harriettehartigan.com, e-mail: H2inA2@aol.com.

p. 130, upper right: Courtesy Dr. Mary Ann Lewis, Professor and Chair of Primary Care Section, University of California-Los Angeles School of Nursing.

p. 130, left: Courtesy Dr. Mary Ann Lewis, Professor and Chair of Primary Care Section, University of California-Los Angeles School of Nursing.

p. 130, center: Courtesy Dr. Mary Ann Lewis, Professor and Chair of Primary Care Section, University of California-Los Angeles School of Nursing.

p. 130, lower right: Courtesy Dr. Mary Ann Lewis, Professor and Chair of Primary Care Section, University of California-Los Angeles School of Nursing.

p. 131, lower left: Courtesy Dr. Mary Ann Lewis, Professor and Chair of Primary Care Section, University of California-Los Angeles School of Nursing.

p. 131, upper left: Courtesy Dr. Mary Ann Lewis, Professor and Chair of Primary Care Section, University of California-Los Angeles School of Nursing.

p. 131, center: Courtesy Dr. Mary Ann Lewis, Professor and Chair of Primary Care Section, University of California-Los Angeles School of Nursing.

p. 131, right: Courtesy Dr. Mary Ann Lewis, Professor and Chair of Primary Care Section, University of California-Los Angeles School of Nursing.

p. 132, left: Courtesy MedStar Health Visiting Nurse Association serving Washington D.C., Maryland, and Northern Virginia.

p. 132, right: Courtesy MedStar Health Visiting Nurse Association serving Washington D.C., Maryland, and Northern Virginia.

p. 133, text: Courtesy Dolores Wright, Loma Linda, California.

159

Within these photos and stories you have shared the many rich journeys of nurses throughout the century. Their love, skill, knowledge, and spirit are the true essence of their work and caring.

Thank you for joining us.

Nurses, thank you for all you do.

THE PUBLISHER

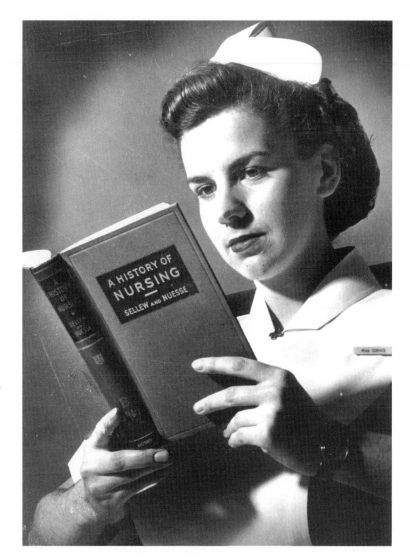